ORIGIN & INSERTION CHARTS
FOR MASSAGE THERAPISTS

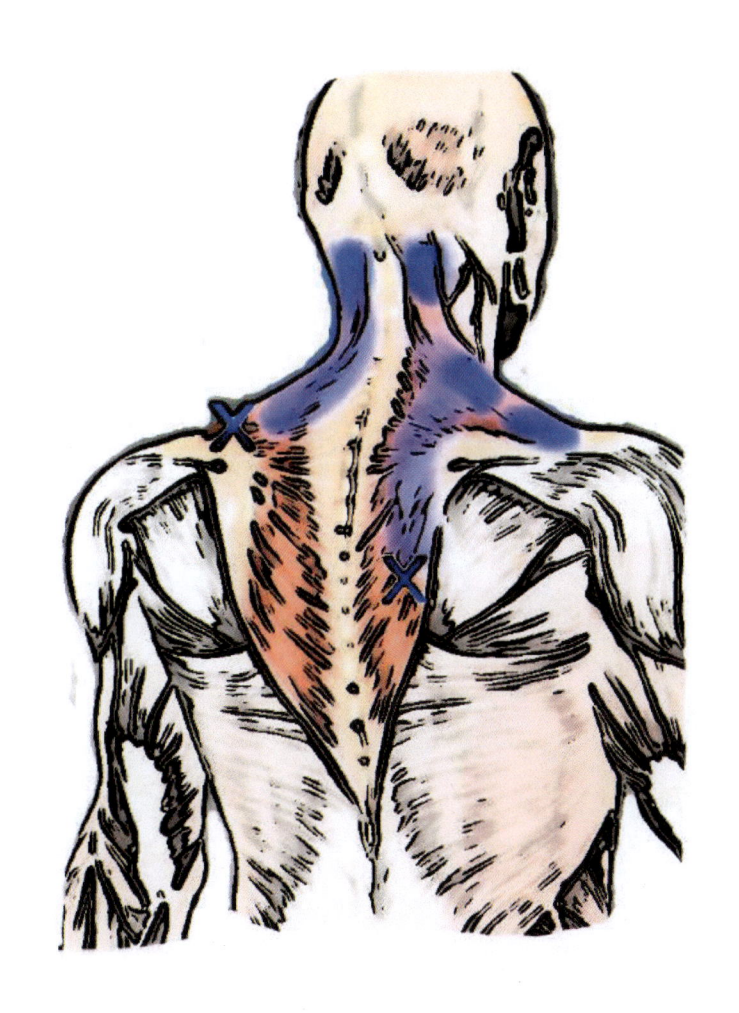

THOMAS VAS-DON

Copyright © 2018 by Thomas Vas-Don
All rights reserved. This book or any portion thereof may not be reproduced or transmitted in any form or manner, electronic or mechanical, including photo copying, printing, recording, or by any information storage or retrieval system, without the express written permission of the copyright owner except for the use of brief quotations in a book review or other noncommercial uses permitted by copyright law.

Revised on
2021

THANK YOU
Thank you to all that believed in me and pushed me to be better. A special thank you to Lynette Jones for bestowing your knowledge and teaching me everything I know.

INTRODUCTION

In this book you will see that the body has been broken down into sections so it is easier to understand when you are studying.

At the first section of this book is the origins and insertions of the muscles in the human body, and as you will see at the back half of the book will be trigger points and pain referral patterns as well as pictures that correspond with the trigger point pain referral pattern charts.

This will be a great book to have when studying and also when you have finished your studies it will be a great book to have a quick reference guide.

Table of Contents

Introduction	1.
Range Of Motion	3.
Orthopaedic testing chart names	5.
Muscles of the Shoulder Girdle	6.
Muscles of the Glenohumeral Joint	8.
Muscles of the Elbow Joint	11.
Muscles of the Hand, Wrist and Thumb	13.
Muscles of the Spine and Abdomen	16.
Muscles of the Pelvis and Hip	19.
Muscles of the Knee	22.
Muscles of the Ankle and Foot	25.
TRIGGER POINT REFERRAL PATERNS	**28.**
Feet and Ankle Referral Pain Chart/Diagrams	29.
Leg Pain Referral Pain Chart/Diagrams	33.
Knee Pain Referral Chart/Diagrams	37.
Thigh Pain Referral Pain Chart/Diagrams	40.
Buttocks Pain Referral Pain Chart/Diagrams	49.
Abdominal Pain Referral Chart/Diagrams	56.
Back Pain Referral Chart/Diagrams	59.
Neck and Shoulder Pain Referral Chart/Diagrams	65.
Arm Pain Referral Chart/Diagrams	74.
Wrist Pain Referral Chart/Diagrams	81.
Anterior Shoulder Pain Chart/diagrams	86.
Headache Pain Referral Chart/diagrams	91.
Orthopaedic Assessments	96.
Abbreviation and Symbols	116.
References	118.

RANGE OF MOTION

(CX) CERVICAL SPINE		
MOVEMENT	RANGE	KEY MUSCLES AFFECTED BY R.O.M
FLEXION	45-50°	Neck extensors and trapezius
EXTENSION	85°	Neck flexors and sternocleidomastoid
LATERAL FLEXION	20-45°	Trapezius, SCM, splenius capitis, longissimus capitis, semispinalis
ROTATION	70-90°	Trapezius, SCM, splenius capitis, obliquus capitis inferior, semispinalis capitis, longissimus capitis

(TX) THORACIC SPINE		
MOVEMENT	RANGE	KEY MUSCLES AFFECTED BY R.O.M
FLEXION	30-40°	Tx Erector spinae, multifidis, rotatores
EXTENSION	0-25°	Rectus abdominis, internal and external obliques, transverse abdominis
LATERAL FLEXION	20-35°	Contralateral Tx erector spinae, contralateral transversospinalis
ROTATION	35-50°	Contralateral Tx erector spinae, ipsilateral transversospinalis

(LX) LUMBAR SPINE		
MOVEMENT	RANGE	KEY MUSCLES AFFECTED BY R.O.M
FLEXION	40-50°	Lx Erector spinae, multifidis, rotatores
EXTENSION	15-30°	Rectus abdominis, internal and external obliques, transverse abdominis
LATERAL FLEXION	25-35°	Contralateral quadartus lumborum, contralateral Lx erector spinae and contralateral transversospinalis
ROTATION	3-20°	Contralateral Lx erector spinae, ipsilateral transversospinalis

HIP and THIGH		
MOVEMENT	RANGE	KEY MUSCLES AFFECTED BY R.O.M
FLEXION	Flexed Knee- 120° Extended Knee- 90°	Hamstrings, gluteus maximus, adductor magnus
EXTENSION	0-15°	Rectus femoris, Iliopsoas
MEDIAL (INTERNAL) ROTATION	0-45°	Adductors, medial, hamstrings
EXTERNAL (LATERAL) ROTATION	0-30°	TFL, gluteus medius, minimus
ABDUCTION	0-40°	Piriformis and the deep external hip rotators
ADDUCTION	0-45°	TFL, gluteus minimus and gluteus medius

KNEE		
MOVEMENT	RANGE	KEY MUSCLES AFFECTED BY R.O.M
FLEXION	0-135°	Quadriceps, TFL (0-30° of flexion)
EXTENSION	0-15°	Hamstrings, gracilis, gastrocnemius, popliteus, plantaris, TFL (in 45-145° of flextion
MEDIAL (INTERNAL) ROTATION	20-30°	Biceps Femoris (non-weight bearing)
LATERAL (EXTERNAL) ROTATION	30-40°	Popliteus, semimembranosus, semitendinosus, Sartorius, gracilis (non- weight)

ANKLE		
MOVEMENT	RANGE	KEY MUSCLES AFFECTED BY R.O.M
PLANTARFLEXION	0-50°	Tibialis anterior, extensor hallicus longus, extensor digitorum longus
DORSIFLEXION	10-20°	Soleus (flexed Knee), gastrocnemius (Knee extended)
INVERSION	45-60°	Peroneus longus, peroneus brevis, extensor digitorum longus
EVERSION	15-30°	Tibialis anterior, tibialis posterior, flexor digitorum longus, flexor hallicus longus, extensor hallicus longus

SHOULDER		
MOVEMENT	RANGE	KEY MUSCLES AFFECTED BY R.O.M
FLEXION	0-180°	Latissimus Dorsi, teres major, sternocostal fibres of pec major, posterior deltoid
EXTENSION	0-50°	Clavicular fibres of pec major, anterior deltoid, biceps brachii
ABDUCTION	0-180°	Latissimus dorsi, teres major, pectoralis (pec) major
ADDUCTION	0-50°	Supraspinatus, deltoid
INTERNAL ROTATION	0-90°	Infraspinatus, teres minor, posterior deltoid
EXTERNAL ROTATION	0-90°	Subscapularis, latissimus dorsi, teres mojor, pec major, anterior deltoid
HORIZONTAL FLEXION (ADDUCTION)	0-140°	Infraspinatus, teres minor, posterior deltoid
HORIZONTAL EXTENTION (ABDUCTION)	0-40°	Pectoralis (pec) major, anterior deltoid

WRIST and ELBOW		
MOVEMENT	RANGE	KEY MUSCLES AFFECTED BY R.O.M
ELBOW FLEXION	140-150°	Triceps Brachii, Anconeus
ELBOW EXTENTION	0-10°	Biceps Brachii, Brachialis, Brachioradialis
FOREARM PRONATION	80-90°	Pronator Teres
FOREARM SUPERNATION	80-90°	Supinator, Biceps Brachii
WRIST FLEXION	80-90°	Common Extensors
WRIST EXTENTION	70-90°	Common flexors

ORTHOPAEDIC TESTING OF THE CERVICAL SPINE (CX)		
MAXIMAL CERVICAL COMPRESSION TEST	CERVICAL DISTRACTION TEST	SHOULDER ABDUCTION TEST (BAKODY'S TEST)
FUNCTIONAL SCREENINIG SEQUENCE		
SCAPULOHUMERAL RHYTHM TEST	NECK FLEXION TEST	PUSH-UP TEST

ORTHOPAEDIC TESTING OF THE THORACIC SPINE (TX)				
ADSON'S TEST	WRIGHT'S TEST	COSTOCLAVICULAR TEST	SLUMP TEST	RESPIRATORY RIB FUNCTION TEST

ORTHOPAEDIC TESTING OF THE LIMBAR SPINE (LX)			
SLUMP TEST	STRAIGHT LEG RAISE TEST (SLR)	PRONE KNEE BEND TEST (NACHLAS')	QUADRANT TEST

ORTHOPAEDIC TESTING OF THE HIP and THIGH		
SLUMP TEST	STRAIGHT LEG RAISE TEST (SLR)	PRONE KNEE BEND TEST (NACHLAS')
THOMAS TEST	OBER'S TEST	TEST FOR SHORT QUADRICEPS
HAMSTRING LENGTH TEST	LONG ADDUCTORS VS SHORT ADDUCTORS	PIRIFORMIS STRETCH TEST

ORTHOPAEDIC TESTING OF THE KNEE		
VARUS/VALGUS STRESS TEST	ANTEROPOSTERIOR DRAWER TEST	McMURRAY'S CLICK TEST
APLEY'S GRIND and DISTRACTION TEST	PATELLOFEMORAL GRINDING TEST (FOUCHET'S SIGN)	PATELLAR APPREHENSION TEST

ORTHOPAEDIC TESTING OF THE ANKLE		
THOMSON'S TEST	ANTERIOR FOOT DRAWER TEST	ANKLE LEATERAL and MEDIAL STABILITY TEST

ORTHOPAEDIC TESTING OF THE SHOULDER		
PECTORALIS MAJOR VS LATISSIMUS DORSI TEST	LATISSIMUS DORSI TRUNK FLEXTION TEST	SUBSCAPULARIS/PECTORLIS MINOR TEST
APLEY'S SCRATCH TEST	SHOULDER ABDUCTION TEST (BAKODY'S)	THE LIFT-OFF TEST
NEER IMPINGEMENT TEST	HAWKINS-KENNEDY IMPINGEMENT TEST	POSTERIOR INTERNAL IMPINGEMENT TEST
EMPTY CAN OR JOBE'S TEST (SUPRASPINATUS TEST)	ACROMIOCLAVICULAR SHEAR TEST	LOAD and SHIFT TEST

ORTHOPAEDIC TESTING OF THE ELBOW and WRIST		
COZENS TEST	MILL'S TEST	LATERAL EPICONDYLE EXTENSION TEST
FLEXOR/PRONATOR TENDINOPATHY TEST	TINEL'S TEST (AT THE ELBOW)	PHALEN'S TEST
TINEL'S SIGN	CARPAL COMPERSSION TEST	FINKELSTEIN'S TEST

MUSCLES OF THE SHOULDER GIRDLE.

| ORIGIN AND INSERTION CHART 1. ||
Muscles	
TRAPEZIUS.	PECTORALIS MINOR.
SERRATUS ANTERIOR.	RHOMBOIDS.
LEVATOR SCAPULAR.	(UF= Upper Fibres, MF= Middle Fibres, LF= Lower Fibres)

ORIGIN AND INSERTION CHART 1.

MUSCLE	ORIGIN	INSERTION	ACTION
Trapezius	Occipital bone, spines of c7 and all thoracic vertebrae	Clavicle, Acromion and spine of scapula	UF= elevate and extends the head MF= adducts scapula LF= depress scapula UP and LF= rotate scapula upwards (medial) and stabilize
Pectoralis Minor	2nd – 5th Rib 3rd -5th or 2nd -4th	Coracoid Process of Scapula	Abducts scapula and rotates it downwards Elevates ribs during forced inhalation
Serratus Anterior (boxer's muscle)	1st -8th/9th Rib	Vertebral/ medial border and inferior angle of scapula	Abducts scapula, rotates upwards (protraction). Elevates ribs when scapula is stabilized
Rhomboid Major	T 2 – T 5	Vertebral/ medial border of scapula	Elevates and adducts (retracts) scapula and rotates downwards Stabilizers of the scapula
Rhomboid Minor	C 7 and T1	Vertebral/ medial border of scapula superior to the spine	Elevates and adducts (retracts) scapula and rotates downwards Stabilizers of the scapula
Levator Scapulae	1st – 4th cervical vertebrae	Medial angle of scapula (between the superior angle and base of spine)	Elevates and adducts (retracts) scapula and rotates downwards Stabilizers of scapula

MUSCLES OF THE GLENOHUMERAL JOINT.

ORIGIN AND INSERTION CHART 2.	
Muscles	
Pectoralis Major	Latissimus Dorsi
Supraspinatus	Infraspinatus
Teres Minor	Teres Major
Deltoid	Subscapularis

ORIGIN AND INSERTION CHART 2.

MUSCLE	ORIGIN	INSERTION	ACTION
Pectoralis Major	Clavicle, sternum and costal cartilage of $2^{nd} - 6^{th}$ ribs	Lip of the intertubercular groove of the humerus (Bicipital groove) Upper fibres anteriorly and inferiorly Lower fibres posteriorly and superiorly	As a whole it adducts and medially rotates. Clavicle head (upper fibres) flexes arm, horizontally adducts shoulder
Latissimus Dorsi	Spinous processes of T6- T12 Lower ¾ ribs Thoracolumbar aponeurosis Posterior iliac crest	Bicipital groove of the humerus	Extends, adducts and medially rotates the arm at the shoulder joint
Teres Major	Inferior angle lower one third of the lateral border of the scapula	Bicipital groove of the humerus	Medially rotates and adducts the arm Stabilizes the head of humerus in the glenoid cavity
Deltoid	Lateral third of clavicle Acromion Spine of scapula	Deltoid tuberosity	Anterior fibres: flex, medially rotate and horizontally adducts shoulder Posterior fibres: extends, laterally rotates and horizontally abducts All: Abducts

MUSCLE	ORIGIN	INSERTION	ACTION
Supraspinatus S	Supraspinous fossa of the scapula	Greater tubercle of the humerus	Assist deltoid in abducting arm at shoulder joint. Stabilizes the head of humerus in the glenoid cavity
Infraspinatus I	Infraspinous fossa of the scapula	Greater tubercle of the humerus	Laterally rotates and adducts the arm at the shoulder. Stabilizes the head of the humerus in the glenoid cavity
Teres Minor T	Upper two thirds of the lateral border of the scapula	Greater tubercle of the humerus	Laterally rotates and adducts the arm. Stabilizes the head of the humerus in the glenoid cavity
Subscapularis S	Subscapular fossa	Lesser tubercle of the humerus	Medially rotates the arm at the shoulder joint and assists in adduction. Stabilizes the head of the humerus in the glenoid cavity

REMEMBER * S. I. T. S* FOR THE ROTATOR CUFF MUSCLES

MUSCLES OF THE ELBOW JOINT

ORIGIN AND INSERTION CHART 3.	
Muscles	
BICEPS BRACHII	BRACHIALIS
BRACHIORADIALIS	TRICEPS
ANCONEUS	SUPINATOR
PRONATOR TERES	PRONATOR QUADRATUS
SH = SHORT HEAD, LH = LONG HEAD, LAT= LATERAL HEAD	

ORIGIN AND INSERTION CHART 3.

MUSCLE	ORIGIN	INSERTION	ACTION
BICEPS BRACHII	**SH**- Coracoid process of scapula **LH** – Supraglenoid tubercle of scapula	Radial tuberosity	Flex elbow, supination Flex the shoulder (GH joint)
BRACHIALIS	Distal half of anterior humerus	Coracoid process of ulna	Flex elbow
BRACHIORADIALIS	Lateral supercondylar ridge	Radial styloid process	Flex elbow (assists in pronation and supination)
TRICEPS	**LH**- infragleneoid tubercle of scapula **LAT H** – Posterior, proximal half of humerus **MH**- Posterior surface distal humerus	Olecranon	**LH**- extends shoulder adducts shoulder **ALL**- extend elbow
ANCONEUS	Lateral epicondyle of the humerus	Olecranon process and superior, posterior ulna	Extend elbow
SUPINATOR	Lateral epicondyle, radial collateral ligament, annular ligament	Anterior lateral surface of radius	Supinates the forearm
PRONATOR TERES	Common flexor tendon from medial epicondyle, coronoid process	Middle of lateral surface of radius	Pronates forearm
PRONATOR QUADRATUS	Medial anterior surface of distal ulna	Lateral anterior surface of distal radius	Pronates forearm

MUSCLES OF THE HAND, WRIST AND THUMB

ORIGIN AND INSERTION CHART 4 & 5.	
Muscles	
EXTENSOR CARPI RADIALIS LONGUS	EXTENSOR CARPI RADIALIS BREVIS
EXTENSOR CARPI ULNARIS	EXTENSOR DIGITORUM
FLEXOR CARPI RADIALIS	FLEXOR CARPI ULNARIS
PALMARIS LONGUS	FLEXOR DIGITORUM SUPERFICIALIS
FLEXOR DIGITORUM PROFUNDUS	
LONG MUSCLES OF THE THUMB	
ABDUCTOR POLLICIS LONGUS	EXTENSOR POLLICIS LONGUS AND BREVIS
FLEXOR POLLICIS LONGUS	
SHORTS MUSCLES OF THE THUMB	
ABDUCTOR POLLICIS BREVIS	OPPENENS POLLICIS
ADDUCTOR POLLICIS	ABDUCTOR DIGITI MINIMI
FLEXOR DIGITI MINIMI BREVIS	OPPENENS DIGITI MINIMI

ORIGIN AND INSERTION CHART 4, 5

MUSCLE	ORIGIN	INSERTION	ACTION
EXTENSOR CARPI RADIALIS LONGUS	Lateral epicondyle of humerus	Base of 2nd metacarpal	Extends the wrist
EXTENSOR CARPI RADIALIS BREVIS	Lateral epicondyle of humerus	Base of metacarpals 2 and 3	Extends and abducts the wrist
EXTENSOR CARPI ULNARIS	Lateral epicondyle of humerus	Base of 5th metacarpal	Extends and adducts the wrist
EXTENSOR DIGITORUM	Lateral epicondyle of humerus	Middle and distal phalanxes of metacarpals 2-5	Extends the fingers and also the wrist
FLEXOR CARPI RADIALIS	Medial epicondyle of humerus	Base of 2nd and 3rd metacarpals	Flex and abducts the wrist (radiocarpal joint) May assist to flex the elbow (humeroulna joint)
FLEXOR CARPI ULNARIS	**Humeral head:** medial epicondyle of humerus **Ulnar head:** proximal two thirds of ulna (ulna shaft)	Pisiform, hook of hamate and base of 5th metacarpal	Flex and adduct the wrist (radiocarpal joint) May assist to flex the elbow (humeroulna joint)
PALMARIS LONGUS	Medial epicondyle of humerus	Flexor retinaculum and palmar aponeurosis	Flex the wrist May assist to flex the elbow (humeroulna joint), tense the palmar fascia
FLEXOR DIGITORUM SUPERFICIALIS	Medial epicondyle of humerus, ulnar collateral ligament, coronoid process interosseous membrane and shaft of radius	Sides of middle phalanges, of 2nd through to 5th fingers	Flex 2nd through to 5th fingers, Flex the wrist
FLEXOR DIGITORUM PROFUNDUS	Anterior and medial surface of ulnar	Base of distal phalanges, palmer surface of 2nd through to 5th fingers	Flex 2nd through to 5th fingers Assists to flex the wrist

LONG MUSCLES OF THE THUMB

MUSCLE	ORIGIN	INSERTION	ACTION
ABDUCTOR POLLLICIS LONGUS	Posterior surface of radius and ulnar and interosseous membrane	Base of 1st metacarpal	Abducts the thumb Extends the thumb Abducts the wrist
EXTENSOR POLLICIS LONGUS and BREVIS	**Longus:** posterior surface of ulnar and interosseous membrane **Brevis:** posterior surface of radius and interosseous membrane	**Longus:** base of distal phalanx of thumb **Brevis:** base of proximal phalanx of thumb	Extends the thumb Abducts the wrist
FLEXOR POLLICIS LONGUS	Anterior surface of radius and interosseous membrane	Base of distal phalanx of thumb	Flex the thumb Assists to flex the wrist

SHORTS MUSCLES OF THE THUMB and 5th DIGIT

MUSCLE	ORIGIN	INSERTION	ACTION
ABDUCTOR POLLICIS BREVIS	**Superficial head:** flexor retinaculum **Deep head:** trapezium, trapezoid and capitate	Base of proximal phalanx of thumb	Flex the thumb Assist in opposition of the thumb
OPPENENS POLLICIS	Flexor retinaculum, Trapezium tubercle	Entire length of the 1st metacarpal bone	Opposition of the thumb at CM joint Brings pads of the thumb and 5th fingers together
ADDUCTOR POLLICIS	Capitate, 2nd and 3rd metacarpals	Base of proximal phalanx of thumb	Adducts the thumb Assists in flexion of the thumb
ABDUCTOR DIGITI MINIMI	Pisiform and tendon of FCU	Base of proximal phalanx of 5th finger	Adducts the 5th finger Assists in opposition of the 5th finger towards the thumb
FLEXOR DIGITI MINIMI BREVIS	Hook of hamate and flexor retinaculum	Base of phalanx of 5th finger	Flex the 5th finger Assists in opposition of the 5th finger towards the thumb
OPPENENS DIGITI MINIMI	Hook of hamate and flexor retinaculum	Shaft of 5th metacarpal, medial surface	Opposition of the 5th finger towards the thumb

MUSCLES OF THE SPINE AND ABDOMEN

ORIGIN AND INSERTION CHART 6.	
Muscles	
ERCTOR SPINAE GROUP	SPINALIS THORACIC
SPINALIS CERVICIS	LONGISSIMUS THORACIS
LONGISSIMUS CERVICIS	LONGISSIMUS CAPITIS
ILIOCOSTALIS LUMBORUM	ILIOCOSTALIS THORACIS
ILIOCOSTALIS CERVICIS	QUADRATUS LUMBORUM
RECTUS ABDOMINIS	EXTERNAL OBLIQUES
INTERNAL OBLIQUES	TRANSVERSE ABDOMINIS
INTERNAL INTERCOSTAL	EXTERNAL INTERCOSTAL
STERNOCLEIDOMASTOID	SCALENES

ORIGIN AND INSERTION CHART 6.

MUSCLE	ORIGIN	INSERTION	ACTION
SPINALIS THORACIC	Spinous process of T11 to L2	Spinous process of T1 to T6	Extends and hyperextends the vertebral column
SPINALIS CERVICIS	Ligamentum nuchae Spinous process of C7	Spinous process of C2 to C7	Extends and hyperextends cervical (neck) portion of vertebral column
LONGISSIMUS THORACIS	Transverse process of L1 to L5	Via two slips of transverse process of T1 to T12 Ribs 3-12	Extends and hyperextends vertebral column (back) Laterally flexes vertebral column to the same side
LONGISSIMUS CERVICIS	Transverse process of T1 to T6	Transverse process C2 to C6	
LONGISSIMUS CAPITIS	Transverse process of T1 to T5 articulating process of C4 to C7	Mastoid process	
ILIOCOSTALIS LUMBORUM	Common tendon, post part of iliac crest and sacrum SP of lower lumber and sacral spine	Insert by six slips into the inferior borders of the lower six ribs and transverse process of L1 to L3	
ILIOCOSTALIS THORACIS	Lower six ribs	Upper six ribs and transverse process of C7	
ILIOCOSTALIS CERVICIS	Upper six ribs	Transverse process of C4 to C7	
QUADRATUS LUMBORUM	Iliolumbar ligament and iliac crest	12th rib and transverse process of L1-4	Laterally flexes the spine Laterally elevates the pelvis Bilaterally- fix the last rib during forced inhalation and exhalation
RECTUS ABDOMINIS	Pubic crest Pubic symphysis	Cartilage of 5th, 6th and 7th ribs and xipoid process	Flex the vertebral column, tilts pelvis posteriorly

EXTERNAL OBLIQUES	External surface of 5th to 12th rib	Anterior part of iliac crest, abdominal aponeurosis to linea alba	**Unilaterally** Laterally flex the vert. column Rotates vert. column to opposite side **Bilaterally** Flex vert. column Compress abdominal contents
INTERNAL OBLIQUES	Iliac crest, inginual ligament, thoracolumbar facia	Lower 3 ribs, abdominal aponeurosis to linea alba	Same as external obliques
TRANSVERSE ABDOMINIS	Iliac crest, inginual ligament, thoracolumbar facia, lower 6th rib	abdominal aponeurosis to linea alba	Compress abdominal contents
INTERNAL INTERCOSTAL	Inferior border of ribs	Superior border of ribs	Elevates ribs
EXTERNAL INTERCOSTAL	Superior border of ribs	Inferior border of ribs	Depresses ribs
STERNOCLEIDOMASTOID	**Sternal head** Sternum (top of manubrium) **Clavicle head** Medial one third of clavicle	Mastoid process	**Unilaterally** Laterally flex head and neck to the same side Rotate head and neck to the same side **Bilaterally** Flex the neck Assists to elevate the rib cage during inhalation
SCALENES	**Anterior scalenes** TP of C3 –C6 (anterior tubercle) **Middle scalenes** TP of C2 – C7 (posterior tubercle **Posterior scalenes** TP of C6 to C7	First rib

(ORIGIN) Posterior tubercle (INSERTION) Second rib | |

MUSCLES OF THE PELVIS AND HIP

| ORIGIN AND INSERTION CHART 7. ||
Muscles	
PSOAS MAJOR	ILIACUS
RECTUS FEMORIS	SARTORIUS
GLUTEUS MAXIMUS	GLUTEUS MEDIUS
GLUTEUS MINIMIS	BICEP FEMORIS
PIRIFORMIS	SEMITENDINOUS
SEMIMEMBRANOSUS	TENSOR FACIA LATA
ADDUCTOR MAGNUS	ADDUCTOR LONGUS
ADDUCTOR BREVIS	PECTINEUS
GRACILLIS	

ORIGIN AND INSERTION CHART 7.

MUSCLE	ORIGIN	INSERTION	ACTION
PSOAS MAJOR	Tps and bodies Lumbar vertebrae	Lesser trochanter	**With origin fixed** Flexes hip **With insertion fixed** Flexes the trunk
ILIACUS	Iliac fossa	Lesser trochanter	Flexes hip Tilts pelvis posteriorly
RECTUS FEMORIS	Aiis	Tibial tuberosity (via patellar and patellar ligament)	Flexes the hip and extends knee
SARTORIUS	Asis	Medial surface of tibia at pes aserine tendon	Flexes, laterally rotates, abducts the hip Flexes the knee Medially rotates flexed knee
GLUTEUS MAXIMUS	Iliac crest, sacrum, coccyx	Gluteal tuberosity (lower fibres) and iliotibial tract (lower fibres)	Extends and laterally rotates thigh Lower fibres adduct the hip
GLUTEUS MEDIUS	Gluteal surface of ilium just below iliac crest	Lateral aspect of the greater trochanter	**All:** fibres abduct the hip **Anterior fibres:** Flex and medially rotate the hip **Posterior fibres:** extend and laterally rotate hip
GLUTEUS MINIMIS	Gluteal surface of ilium between the anterior and inferior gluteal lines	Anterior aspect of greater trochanter	Abduct, flex, medially rotates hip
BICEP FEMORIS	**Long head:** ischial tuberosity **Short head:** lateral lip of linea aspera	Head of fibula	**Long head:** extends and assists to laterally rotate the hip Tilts pelvis posteriorly
PIRIFORMIS	Lateral surface of sacrum	Greater trochanter of femur	Rotates thigh laterally when hip is extended

MUSCLE	ORIGIN	INSERTION	ACTION
SEMITENDINOUS	Ischial tuberosity	Proximal, medial shaft of tibia at pes anserine	Extends and assists to medially rotate the hip Tilts the pelvis posteriorly
SEMIMEMBRANOSUS	Ischial tuberosity	Posterior aspect of medial condyle of tibia	As above
TENSOR FACIA LATA	Iliac crest posterior to Asis	Iliotibital band (ITB)	Abducts, flexes and medially rotates the hip
ADDUCTOR MAGNUS	Inferior ramus of pubis ramus of ischium and ischial tuberosity	Medial lip of linea aspera and adductor tubercle	**All adductors:** Adduct and medially rotate the hip **except gracillis** **Posterior fibres:** extend hip
ADDUCTOR LONGUS	Pubic tubercle	Medial lip of linea aspera	As above
ADDUCTOR BREVIS	Inferior ramus of pubis	Pectineal line and medial lip of linea aspera	As above
PECTINEUS	Superior ramus of pubis	Pectineal line	As above
GRACILLIS	Inferior ramus of pubis	Proximal, medial surface of tibia at pes anserine	Assist to flex the hip Flexes and medially rotates the knee

MUSCLES OF THE KNEE

ORIGIN AND INSERTION CHART 8.	
Muscles	
RECTUS FEMORIS	VASTUS LATERALIS
VASTUS MEDIALIS	VASTUS INTERMEDIUS
BICEP FEMORIS	SEMITENDINOUS
SEMIMEMBRANOSUS	GRACILLIS
SARTORIUS	GASTROCNEMIS
POPLITEUS	PLANTARIS

ORIGIN AND INSERTION CHART 8.

MUSCLE	ORIGIN	INSERTION	ACTION
RECTUS FEMORIS	Aiis	Tibial tuberosity (via patella tendon)	All 4 heads extend the leg at the knee joint
VASTUS LATERALIS	Lateral lip of linea aspera Gluteal tuberosity and greater trochanter	As above	As above
VASTUS MEDIALIS	Medial lip of linea aspera	As above	As above
VASTUS INTERMEDIUS	Anterior and lateral shaft of femur	As above	As above
BICEP FEMORIS	**Long head:** ischial tuberosity **Short head:** lateral lip of linea aspera	Head of fibula	**Long head:** extends and assists to laterally rotate the hip Tilts pelvis posteriorly Flex and laterally rotates flexed knee
SEMITENDINOUS	Ischial tuberosity	Proximal, medial shaft of tibia at pes anserine	Extends and assists to medially rotate the hip Tilts the pelvis posteriorly
SEMIMEMBRANOSUS	Ischial tuberosity	Posterior aspect of medial condyle of tibia	As above
GRACILLIS	Inferior ramus of pubis	Proximal, medial surface of tibia at pes anserine	Assist to flex the hip Flexes and medially rotates the knee
SARTORIUS	Asis	Medial surface of tibia at pes aserine tendon	Flexes, laterally rotates, abducts the hip Flexes the knee Medially rotates flexed knee
GASTROCNEMIS	Condyles of femur posterior surface	Calcaneus via the calcaneus tendon (Achilles tendon)	Flex the knee

POPLITEUS	Lateral condyle of the femur	Proximal, posterior aspect of tibia	Medially rotates flexed knee, flexed the knee, medially rotates the tibia to unlock the extended knee
MUSCLE	**ORIGIN**	**INSERTION**	**ACTION**
PLANTARIS	Lateral supracondylar line of femur	Calcaneus via the calcaneus tendon (Achilles tendon)	Weak flexion of the knee

BURSAE	
Suprapatellar	Prepatella
Infrapatellar	Infrapatellar fat pad

MUSCLES OF THE ANKLE AND FOOT

ORIGIN AND INSERTION CHART 9.	
Muscles	
TIBIALIS ANTERIOR	EXTENSOR HALLUCIS LONGUS
EXTENSOR DIGITORUM LONGUS	PERONEUS TERTIUS
PERONEUS LONGUS	PERONEUS BREVIS
FLEXOR DIGITORUM LONGUS	FLEXOR HALLUCIS LONGUS
TIBIALIS POSTERIOR	GASTROCNEMIS
SOLEUS	EXTENSOR DIGITORUM BREVIS
FLEXOR DIGITORUM BREVIS	ABDUCTOR DIGITI MINIMI
ABDUCTOR HALLUCIS	

MUSCLE	ORIGIN	INSERTION	ACTION
TIBIALIS ANTERIOR	Lateral condyle of tibia; proximal, lateral surface of tibia and interosseous membrane	Under surface of cuneiform and the base of the 1st metacarpal	Inverts foot Dorsi flexes the ankle
EXTENSOR HALLUCIS LONGUS	Middle anterior surface of the fibula and interosseous membrane	Base of the distal phalanx of the 1st toe	Extends the 1st toe Dorsi flexes the ankle Inverts the foot
EXTENSOR DIGITORUM LONGUS	Lateral condyle of tibia; proximal, anterior shaft of fibula and interosseous membrane	Middle and distal phalanges of 2nd through to 5th toes	Extends the 2nd through to 5th toes Dorsi flexes the ankle Inverts the foot
PERONEUS TERTIUS	Anterior fibula interosseous membrane	5th metatarsal	Dorsi flexes foot at ankle Everts foot
PERONEUS LONGUS	Head and upper two thirds of the lateral surface of the fibula	Crosses the foot to insert into plantar and lateral surface of the medial cuneiform and base of the 1st metatarsal	Everts foot Assists to flex the ankle
PERONEUS BREVIS	Distal two thirds of lateral surface of the fibula	Tuberosity of the 5th metatarsal	Enverts foot Assists plantar flex the ankle
FLEXOR DIGITORUM LONGUS	Middle posterior surface of the tibia	Runs along the sole of the foot -divides into 4 tendons - inserts into the base of the distal phalanges of 2nd through 5th toe	Flex 2nd-5th toes Weak plantar flex the ankle Inverts the foot
FLEXOR HALLUCIS LONGUS	Middle half of posterior surface of the fibula	Runs along the sole of the foot -inserts into plantar base of distal phalanx of the big toe	Flex the 1st toe Weak plantar Flex the ankle Inverts the foot
TIBIALIS POSTERIOR	Proximal posterior shaft of tibia and fibula Posterior surface of the interosseous membrane	All 5 tarsals bone and bases of 2nd through to 4th metatarsal	Invert the foot Plantar flex the ankle
GASTROCNEMIS	Condyles of femur posterior surface	Calcaneus via the calcaneus tendon (Achilles tendon)	Flex the knee Plantar flex the ankle

MUSCLE	ORIGIN	INSERTION	ACTION
SOLEUS	Back part of the head of the fibula -upper posterior part of the shaft of the fibula -soleal line of tibia Posterior surface of tibia	Calcaneus via the calcaneus tendon (Achilles tendon)	Plantar flex the ankle
EXTENSOR DIGITORUM BREVIS	Dorsal surface of calcaneus	2nd through 4th toes via the extensor digitorum longus tendon	Extends the 2nd – 4th toes (metatarsophalangeal and interphalangeal joints)
FLEXOR DIGITORUM BREVIS	Medial process of calcaneus and plantar aponeurosis	Middle phalanges of 2nd -5th toes	Flex middle phalanges of the 2nd – 5th toes
ABDUCTOR DIGITI MINIMI	Lateral process of calcaneus and plantar aponeurosis	Proximal phalanx of 5th toe (lateral surface)	Flex the 5th Assist to abduct the 5th toe
ABDUCTOR HALLUCIS	Medial process of calcaneus and plantar aponeurosis	Proximal phalanx of 1st toe (medial surface) and medial sesamoid bone	Abduct the first toe Assist to flex the 1st toe

ORIGIN AND INSERTION CHART 9.

TRIGGER POINT REFERRAL PATTERNS

CHARTS AND PICTURES

Book compiled by Thomas Vas-Don.

Illustrations by Daniel Thomas.

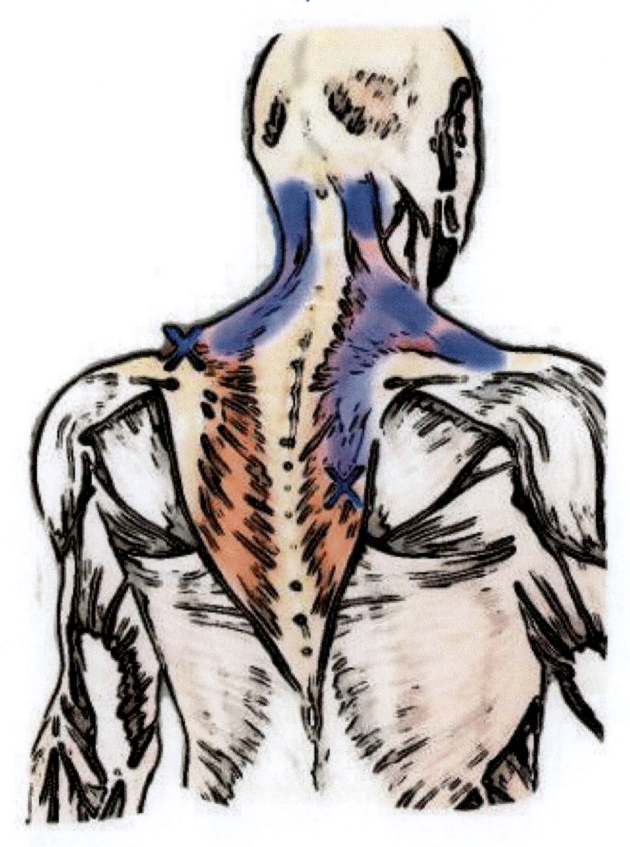

FEET AND ANKLE REFERRAL PAIN CHART / DIAGRAMS

Location of Pain	Muscle	Referral	Picture Ref no:
Anterior Ankle Pain	Tibialis Anterior	The anterior aspect of the ankle, the big toe and the dorsal part of the foot and up into the anterior lower leg.	Ref no: 1
Anterior Ankle Pain	Peroneus Tertius	Pain and tenderness along the anterior and lateral aspect of the ankle, with some overflow to the posterior side of the Malleolus.	Ref no: 2
Anterior Ankle Pain	Extensor Digitorium Longus	Pain referring into the Dorsal aspect of the foot and middle three toes, which will refer up the lower leg.	Ref no: 3
Plantar of Foot Pain	Gastrocnemius	Most common trigger point in the middle of the belly of the muscle which refers pain into the instep of the foot, which spread throughout the entire posterior lower leg. The next common point is the lateral head, which refers pain around itself. The other two points are near the attachment sites into the Femur, and will refer pain into the posterior knee. NOTE: The two trigger point locations in the muscle belly can cause nocturnal calf cramps	Ref no: 4
Plantar of Foot Pain	Flexor Digitorium Longus	Refer pain primarily into the middle of the plantar surface of the foot, which can spread to the toes.	Ref no: 5
Plantar of Foot Pain	Abductor Hallucis	Along the medial aspect of the ankle, which spills over into the instep. This can be distinguished from the SOLEUS referral pattern which covers the entire posterior and bottom aspect of the heel. NOTE: Trigger points of this muscle also cause's foot cramps.	Ref no: 6
Plantar of Foot Pain	Soleus	Distal trigger points refer down into the posterior and plantar surface of the ankle. Proximal trigger points refer into the posterior calf. The rarest trigger point in the distal lateral part of the muscle may refer pain into the sacrum.	Ref no: 7
Plantar of Foot Pain	Tibialis Posterior	The primary referral is over the Achilles tendon, which will go down the entire calf and plantar surface of the foot	Ref no: 8

Heel Pain	Abductor Hallucis	Along the medial aspect of the ankle and also into the instep. Which can be distinguished from the SOLEUS referral pattern which covers the entire posterior and bottom aspect of the heel. NOTE: Trigger points of this muscle also cause's foot cramps.	Ref no: 9
Heel Pain	Soleus	Distal trigger points refer down into the posterior and plantar surface of the ankle. Proximal trigger points can refer into the posterior calf. The rarest trigger point in the distal lateral part of the muscle may refer pain into the sacrum.	Ref no: 10
Heel Pain	Tibialis Posterior	The primary referral pattern is over the Achilles tendon, which leads down to the entire calf and plantar surface of the foot	Ref no: 11
Heel Pain	Peroneus Longus and Brevis	Both of these muscles can refer pain to the lateral ankle. But the Peroneus Longus has a small area on the lateral leg. These muscles can frequently have trigger points in cases of ankle instability due to lateral ankle sprains	Ref no: 12

FEET & ANKLE PAIN DIAGRAMS

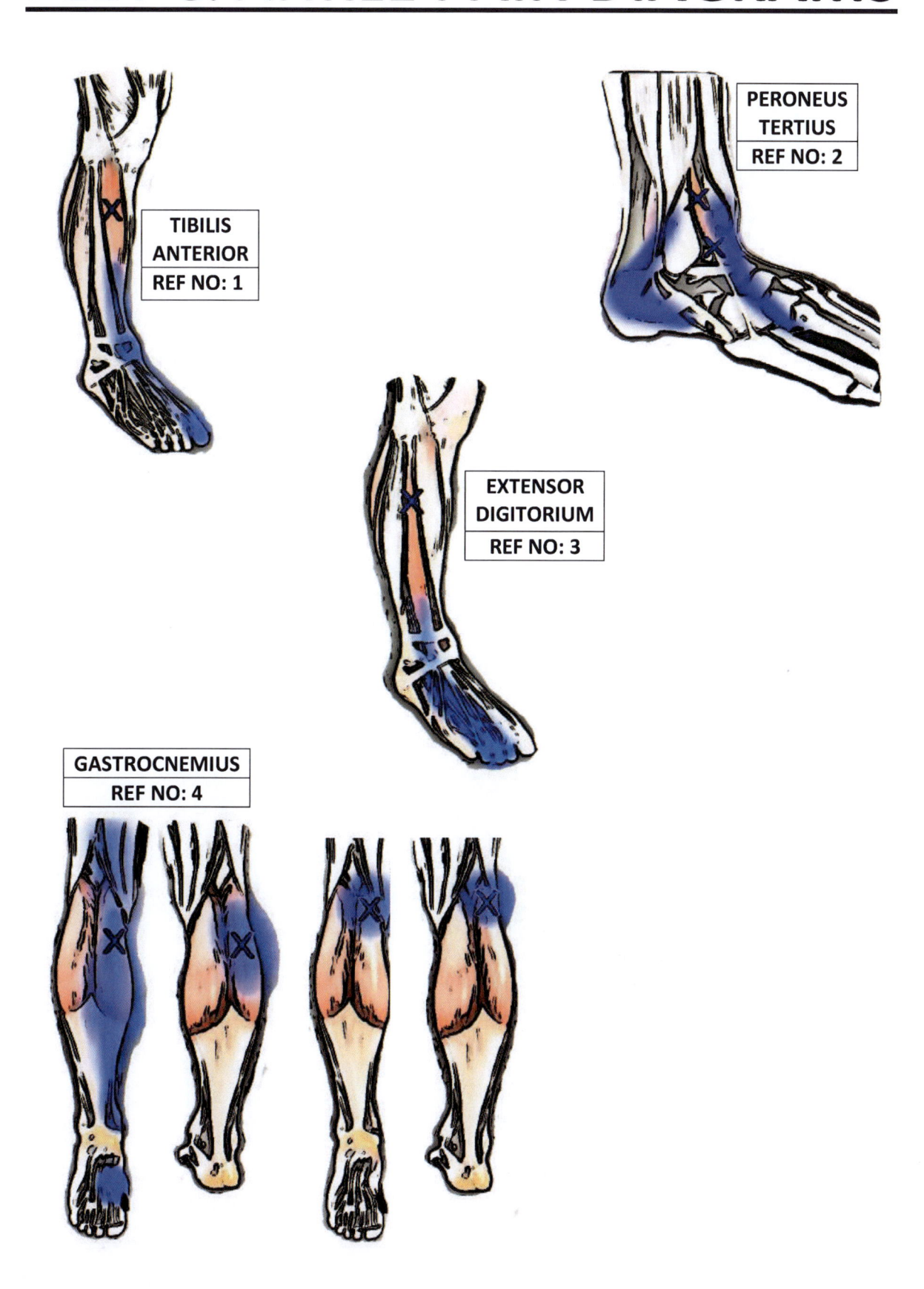

TIBILIS ANTERIOR
REF NO: 1

PERONEUS TERTIUS
REF NO: 2

EXTENSOR DIGITORIUM
REF NO: 3

GASTROCNEMIUS
REF NO: 4

FLEXOR DIGITORIUM
REF NO: 5

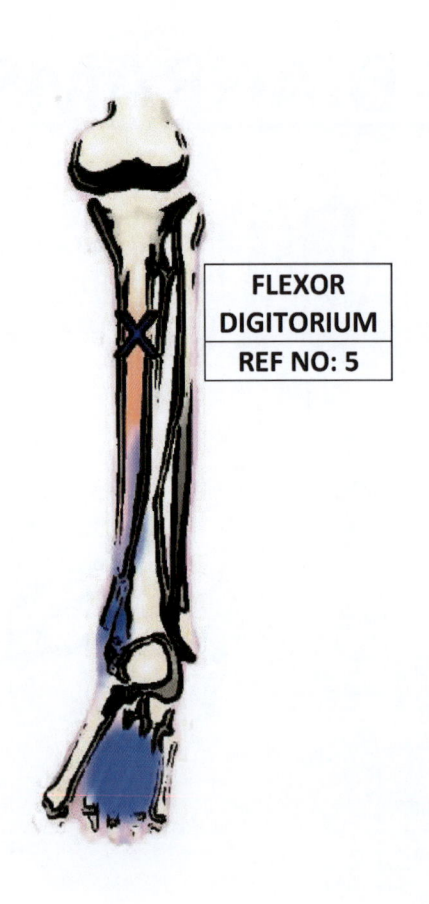

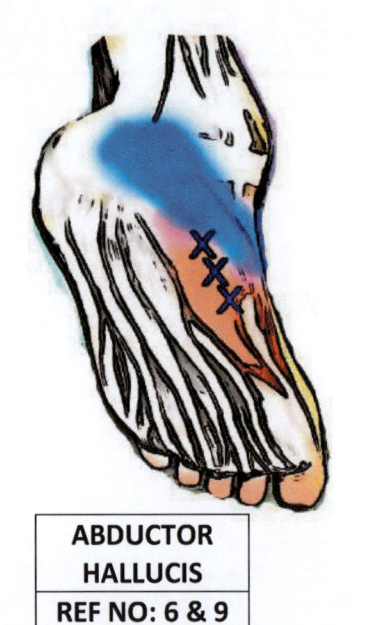

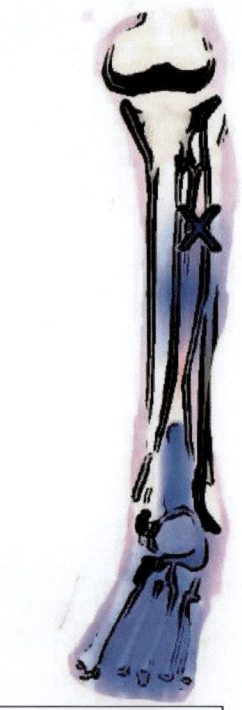

ABDUCTOR HALLUCIS
REF NO: 6 & 9

TIBIALIS POSTERIOR
REF NO: 8 & 11

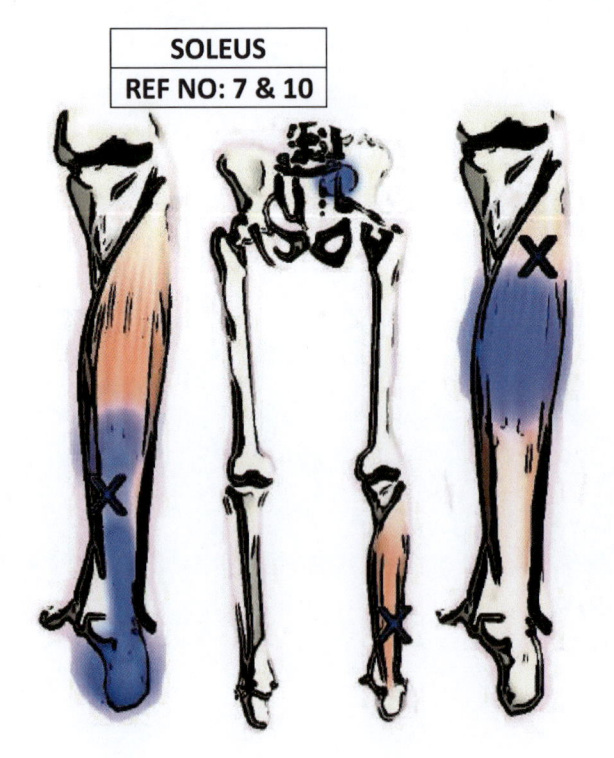

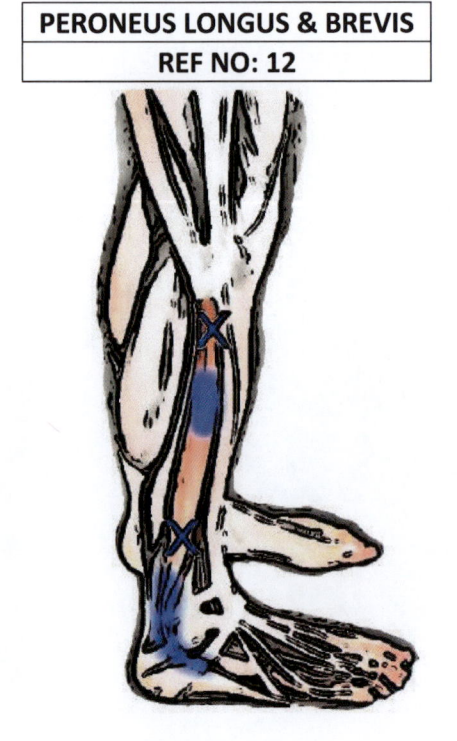

SOLEUS
REF NO: 7 & 10

PERONEUS LONGUS & BREVIS
REF NO: 12

LEG PAIN REFERRAL CHART / DIAGRAMS

Location of Pain	Muscle	Referral	Picture Ref no:
Posterior Leg Pain	Flexor Digitorium Longus	Refers pain primarily into the middle of the plantar surface of the foot, and to the outer of the toes.	Ref no: 1
Posterior Leg Pain	Gastrocnemius	Most common trigger point in the middle of the belly can refer pain into the instep of the foot. Which goes throughout the entire posterior lower leg. Next common point is the lateral head, which will refer pain around itself. The other two points are near the attachment sites into the Femur, and will refer pain into the posterior aspect of the knee. NOTE: The two trigger point locations of this muscle belly can cause nocturnal calf cramps	Ref no: 2
Posterior Leg Pain	Soleus	Distal trigger points refer pain down into the posterior and plantar surface of the ankle. The proximal trigger points refer pain into the posterior calf, and the rarest trigger point is in the distal lateral part of the muscle which may refer pain into the sacrum.	Ref no: 3
Posterior Leg Pain	Tibialis Posterior	The primary referral patter is over the Achilles tendon, which goes down the entire calf and plantar surface of the foot	Ref no: 4
Posterior Leg Pain	Gluteus Minimus	The trigger points in the Anterior portion of this muscle can refer down the lateral leg and into the buttock. The trigger points in the Posterior aspect of this muscle have a similar referral pattern but is more of a posterior referral pattern that does not go all the way down the leg. This referral pattern of this muscle can mimics Sciatica, this muscle should be the first place to be checked. If the straight leg test turns out negative.	Ref no: 5

Posterior Leg Pain	Semitendinosus and Semimembranosus	This main referral pattern goes up into the Gluteal fold, which will/can go all along the posterior leg.	Ref no: 6
Posterior Leg Pain	Gastrocnemius	The most common trigger point is in the middle of the belly of the muscle which refers pain into the instep of the foot which spreads throughout the entire posterior part of the lower leg. The next common trigger point is the lateral head, which refers pain around itself. The other two points are near the attachment sites into the Femur, and will refer pain into the posterior knee. NOTE: The two trigger point locations in the muscle belly can cause nocturnal calf cramps	Ref no: 7
Lateral Leg Pain	Peroneus Longus and Brevis	Both muscles refer to the lateral ankle, but the Peroneus Longus has a small spillover area on the lateral leg. These muscles frequently harbor trigger points in cases of ankle instability due to lateral ankle sprain	Ref no: 8
Lateral Leg Pain	Gluteus Minimus	Trigger points in the Anterior portion of this muscle refer down the lateral leg and into the buttock. Trigger points in the Posterior part of this muscle have a similar but more posterior referral pattern that does not go as far down the leg. Since the referral pattern of this muscle mimics Sciatica, this muscle should be first to be checked for involvement if the straight leg test turns out negative.	Ref no: 9
Lateral Leg Pain	Vastus Lateralis	Superficial trigger points in this muscle refer locally, whereas deeper trigger points have a referral pattern that travels. Deep trigger points in the middle of the muscle refer all along the lateral thigh. Trigger points in distal part of the muscle can refer into the lateral knee. NOTE: This is the largest muscle in the Quadraceps group	Ref no: 10

LEG PAIN CHART DIAGRAMS

FLEXOR DIGITORIUM LONGUS
REF NO: 1

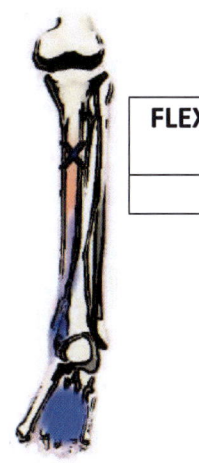

GASTROCNEMIUS
REF NO: 2 & 7

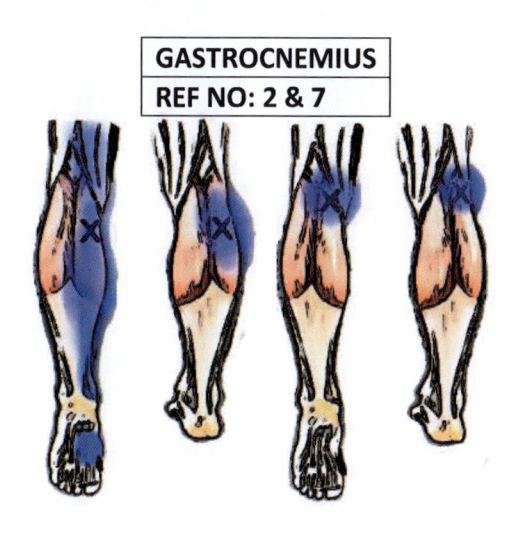

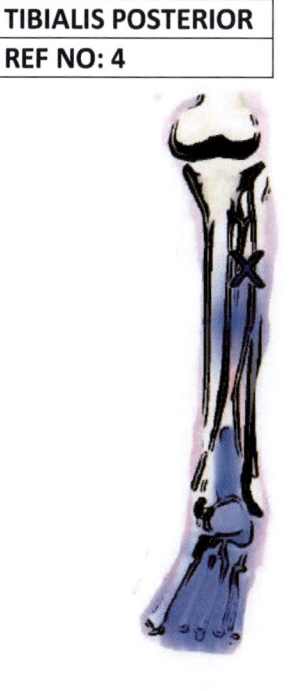

SOLEUS
REF NO: 3

TIBIALIS POSTERIOR
REF NO: 4

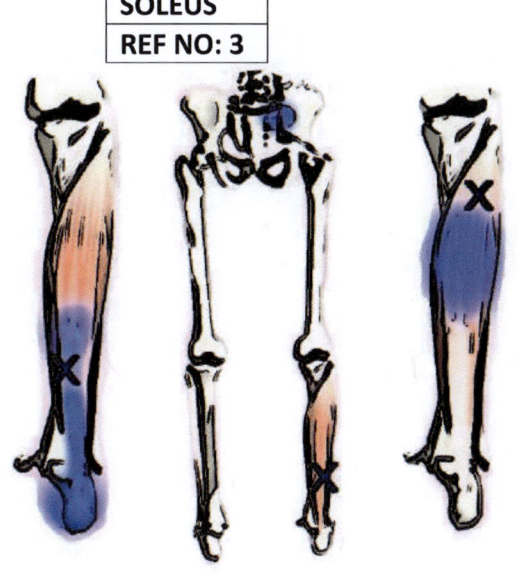

GLUTEUS MINIMUS
REF NO: 5 & 9

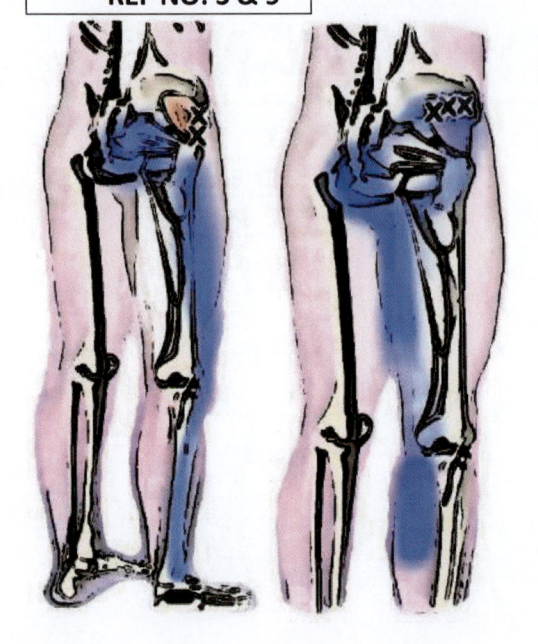

SEMITENDINOSUS & SEMIMEMBRANOSUS
REF NO: 6

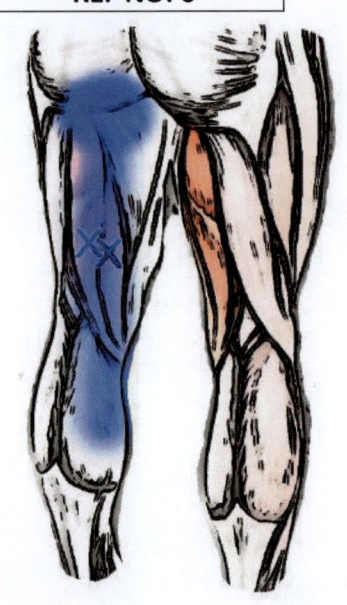

VASTUS LATERALIS
REF NO: 10

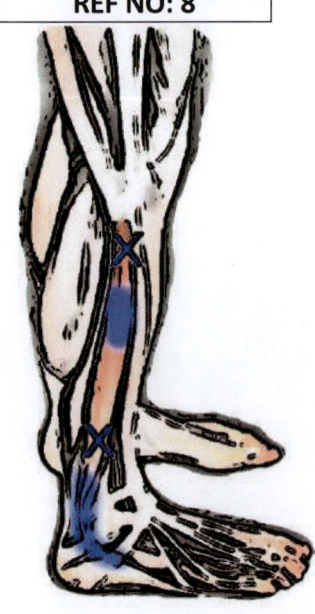

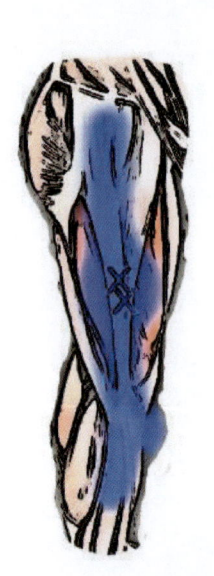

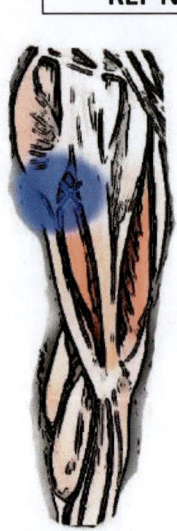

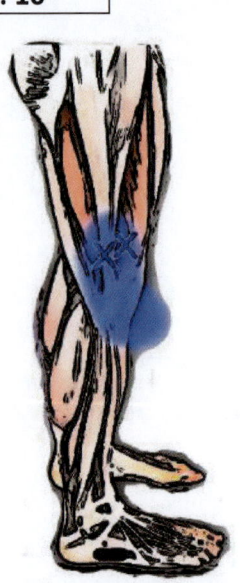

PERONEUS LONGUS & BREVIS
REF NO: 8

KNEE PAIN REFERRAL CHART/ DIAGRAMS

Location of Pain	Muscle	Referral	Picture Ref no:
Anterior Knee Pain	Rectus Femoris	The trigger points high up in the thigh refer down into the knee, with spillover into the anterior thigh	Ref no:1
Anterior Knee Pain	Vastus Medialis	Distal trigger points refer into the anterior medial knee. Proximal trigger points refer along the inner thigh.	Ref no:2
Anterior Knee Pain	Adductor Brevis and Longus	The distal trigger points tend to refer to the upper medial knee, with spillover down the tibia. The more proximal trigger points refer to the anterior hip area.	Ref no: 3
Posterior Knee Pain	Gastrocnemius	Most common trigger point on the middle of the belly of the muscle refers pain into the instep of the foot with spillover throughout the entire posterior lower leg. Next common point is the lateral head, which refers pain around itself. The other two points are near the attachment sites into the Femur, and refer pain into the posterior knee. NOTE: The two trigger point locations in the muscle belly can cause nocturnal calf cramps	Ref no: 4
Posterior Knee Pain	Soleus	Distal trigger points refer down into the posterior and plantar surface of the ankle. Proximal trigger points refer into the posterior calf. The rarest trigger point in the distal lateral part of the muscle may refer pain into the sacrum.	Ref no: 5
Posterior Knee Pain	Semitendinosus and Semimembranosus	The main referral is up into the Gluteal fold, with spillover all along posterior leg.	Ref no: 6
Posterior Knee Pain	Biceps Femoris	The primary referral is the posterior-lateral knee and is experienced as a deep aching. Spillover patterns run into the posterior-lateral thigh.	Ref no: 7
Posterior Knee Pain	Popliteus	Trigger points refer to the back of the knee	Ref no: 8

KNEE PAIN CHART DIAGRAMS

RECTUS FEMORIS
REF NO: 1

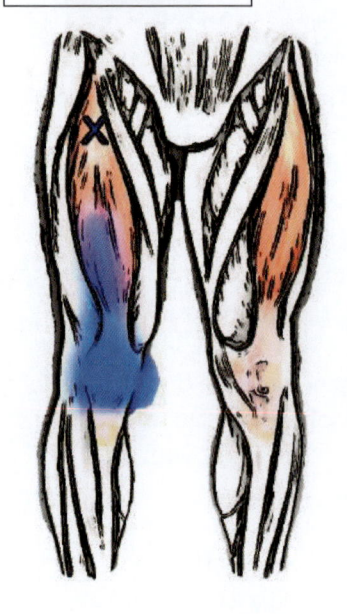

VASTUS MEDIALIS
REF NO: 2

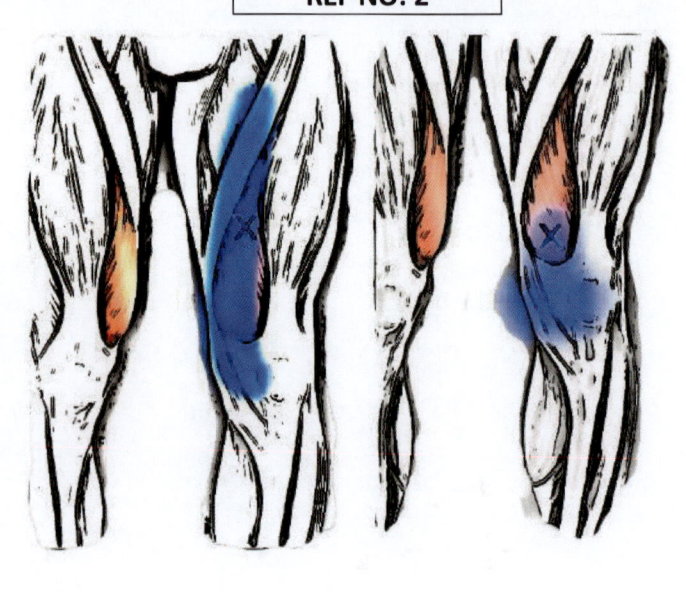

ADDUCTOR BREVIS & LONGUS
REF NO: 3

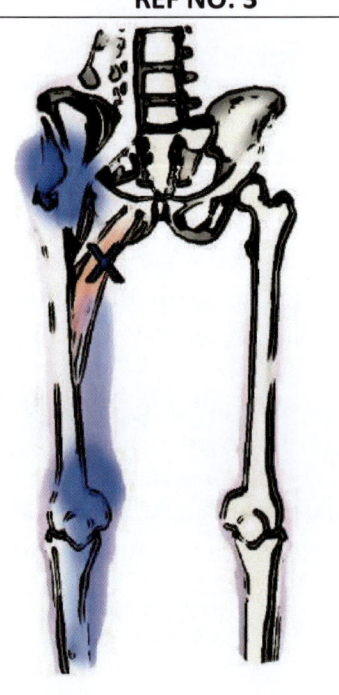

GASTROCNEMIUS
REF NO: 4

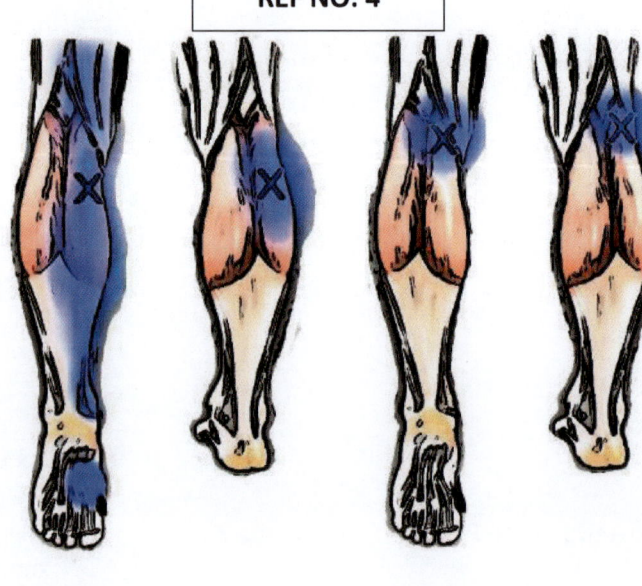

SOLEUS
REF NO: 5

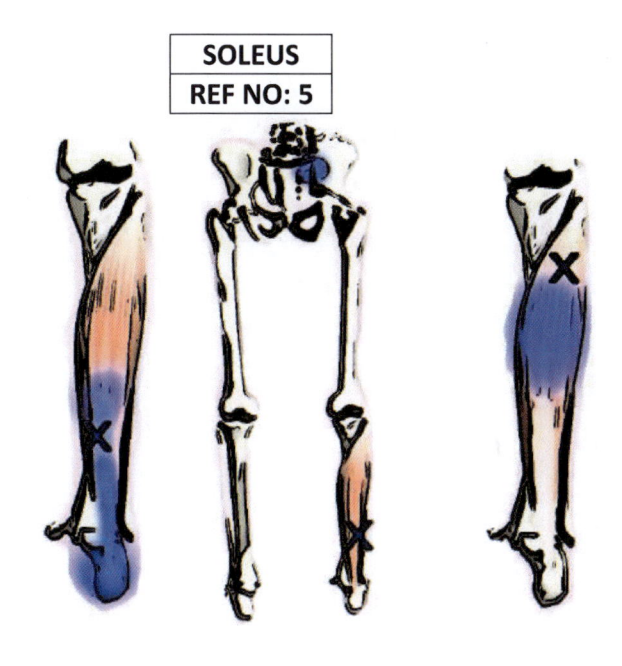

SEMITENDINOSUS & SEMIMEMBRANOSUS
REF NO: 6

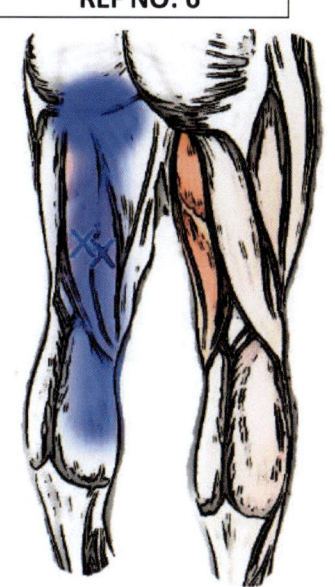

BICEPS FEMORIS
REF NO: 7

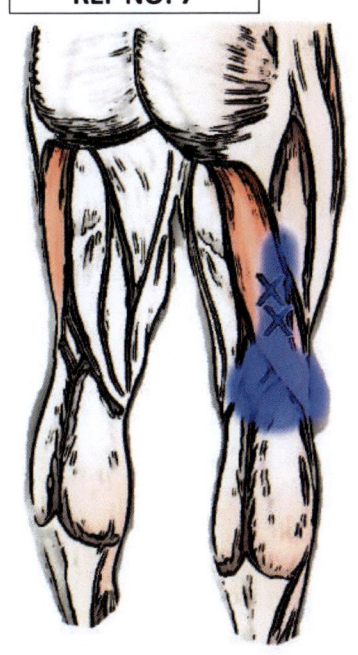

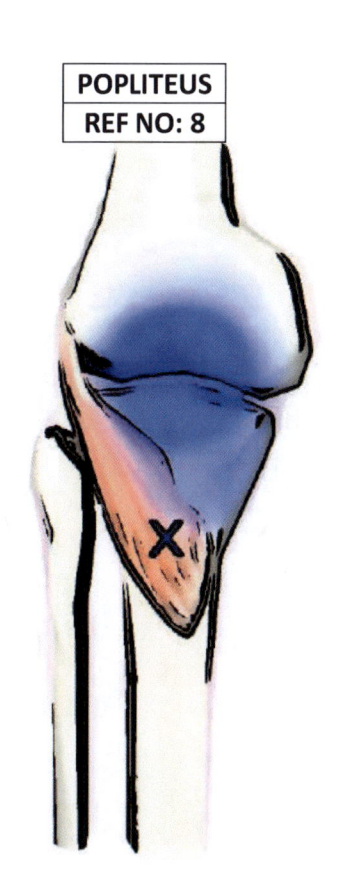

POPLITEUS
REF NO: 8

THIGH PAIN REFERRAL CHART / DIAGRAMS

Location of Pain	Muscle	Referral	Picture Ref no:
Lateral Thigh Pain, Posterior Thigh Pain	Gluteus Minimus	Trigger points in the Anterior portion of this muscle refer down the lateral leg and into the buttock. Trigger points in the Posterior part of this muscle have a similar but more posterior referral pattern that does not go as far down the leg. Since the referral pattern of this muscle mimics Sciatica, this muscle should be first to be checked for involvement if the straight leg test turns out negative.	Ref no: 1
Lateral Thigh Pain	Vastus Lateralis	Superficial trigger points in the muscle refer locally, whereas the deeper trigger points have a referral pattern that travels. Deep trigger points in the middle of the muscle refer all along the lateral thigh. Trigger points in distal part of the muscle can refer into the lateral knee. NOTE: This is the largest muscle in the Quadraceps group	Ref no: 2
Lateral Thigh Pain	Rectus Femoris	The trigger points high up in the thigh refer down into the knee, with spillover into the anterior thigh	Ref no: 3
Lateral Thigh Pain, Posterior Thigh Pain	Piriformis	Trigger points refer pain into the sacro-iliac region, across the posterior hip, and down the thigh	Ref no: 4
Lateral Thigh Pain	Quadratus Lumborum	The uppermost trigger points refer pain to the SI joint and the lateral hip. The most inferior points refer to the buttock. The middle trigger point refer over the SI joint. Some people report a jolting pain to the anterior thigh from deep QL trigger points.	Ref no: 5

Lateral Thigh Pain	Tensor Fasciae Latae	Pain down the lateral aspect of the leg, concentrating over the greater trochanter	Ref no: 6
Lateral Thigh Pain, Anterior Thigh Pain	Vastus Intermedius	Trigger points refer pain downward over the thigh. Occasionally the pain will spread upward.	Ref no: 7
Lateral Thigh Pain	Gluteus Maximus	The trigger points near the sacrum refer pain in a crescent pattern from the sacrum down to the gluteal fold. The most common trigger point location is at the distal portion of the muscle, and refers to the entire buttock, and also deep into the buttock, which can lead to the false conclusion that deeper muscles are involved. The third trigger point lies on the most medial and inferior fibers, next to the coccyx.	Ref no: 8
Anterior Thigh Pain	Rectus Femoris	The trigger points high up in the thigh refer down into the knee, with spillover into the anterior thigh	Ref no: 9
Anterior Thigh Pain	Adductor Brevis and Longus	The distal trigger points tend to refer to the upper medial knee, with spillover down the tibia. The more proximal trigger points refer to the anterior hip area.	Ref no: 10
Anterior Thigh Pain	Psoas and Iliacus	Primarily to the lower lumbar area and sacrum, and secondly to the anterior thigh	Ref no: 11
Anterior Thigh Pain, Inner Thigh Pain	Sartorius	Trigger points in this muscle refer locally with a superficial sharp and tingling pain.	Ref no: 12
Anterior Thigh Pain, Inner Thigh Pain	Pectineus	The referral pattern for this muscle is right around the trigger point on the anterior hip, just inferior to the inguinal ligament The lower trigger points refer to the anterior/inner thigh. The upper points refer pain deep within the pelvis	Ref no: 13
Anterior Thigh Pain, Inner Thigh Pain	Adductor Magnus	The lower trigger points refer to the anterior/inner thigh. The upper points refer pain deep within the pelvis.	Ref no: 14

Inner Thigh Pain	Vastus Medialis	Distal trigger points refer into the anterior medial knee. Proximal trigger points refer along the inner thigh	Ref no: 15
Inner Thigh Pain	Gracilis	Trigger points in the Gracilis produce a local hot, stinging, superficial pain that travels up and down along the inner thigh	Ref no: 16
Posterior Thigh Pain	Semitendinosus and Semimembranosus	The main referral is up into the Gluteal fold, with spillover along the posterior leg.	Ref no: 17
Posterior Thigh Pain	Biceps Femoris	The primary referral is the posterior-lateral knee and is experienced as a deep aching. Spillover patterns run into the posterior-lateral thigh.	Ref no: 18
Posterior Thigh Pain	Obturator Internus	The main referral pattern is into the coccyx, with less common referral down the posterior thigh	Ref no: 19

THIGH PAIN CHART DIAGRAMS

GLUTEUS MINIMUS
REF NO: 1

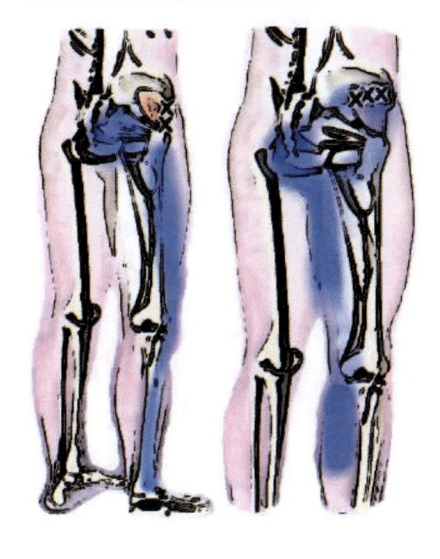

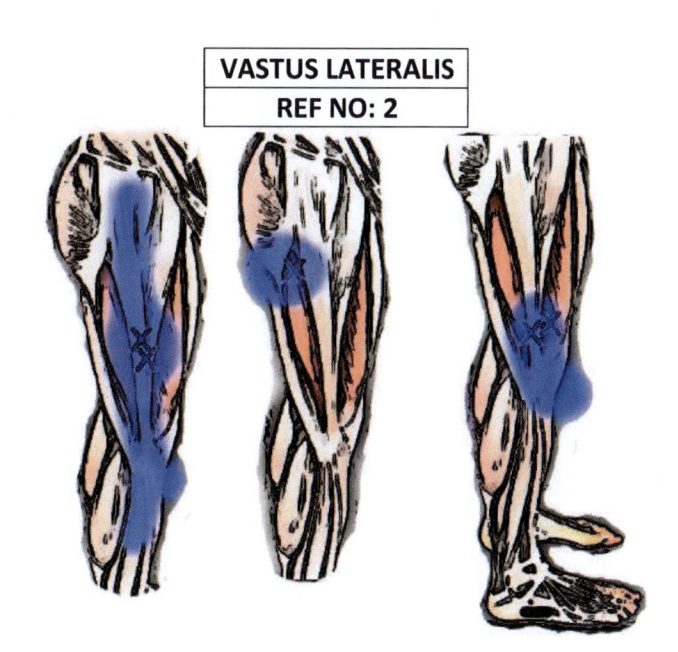

VASTUS LATERALIS
REF NO: 2

RECTUS FEMORIS
REF NO: 3 & 9

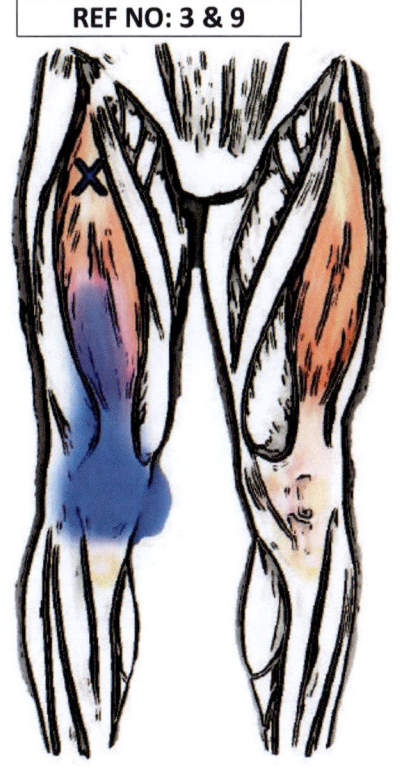

PIRIFORMIS
REF NO: 4

QUADRATUS LUMBORUM
REF NO: 5

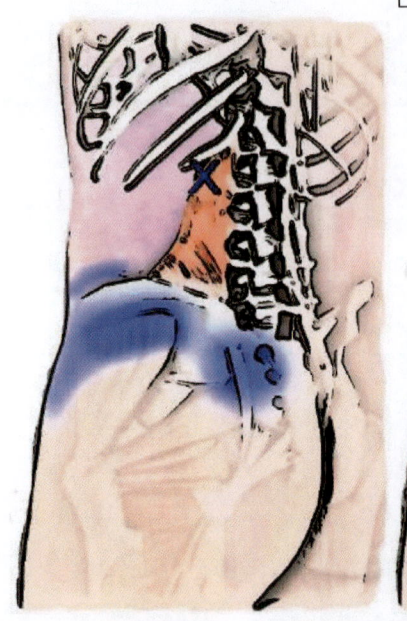

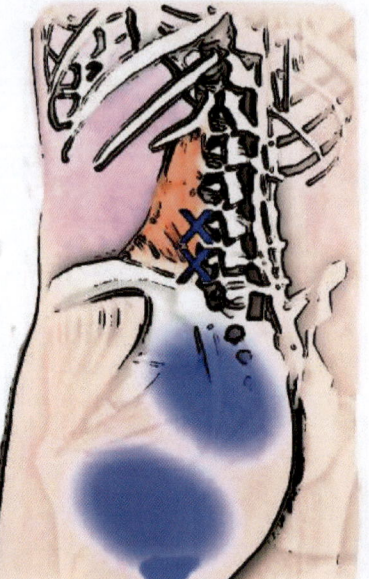

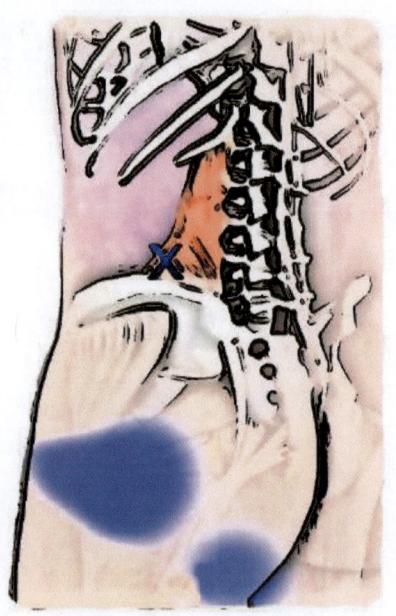

TFL
REF NO: 6

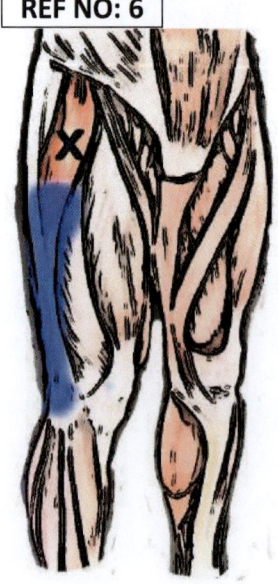

VASTUS INTERMEDIUS
REF NO:7

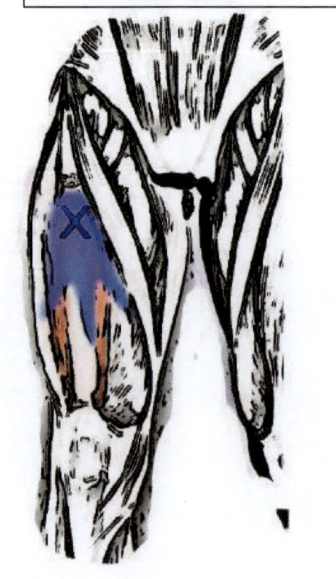

GLUTEUS MAX
REF NO: 8

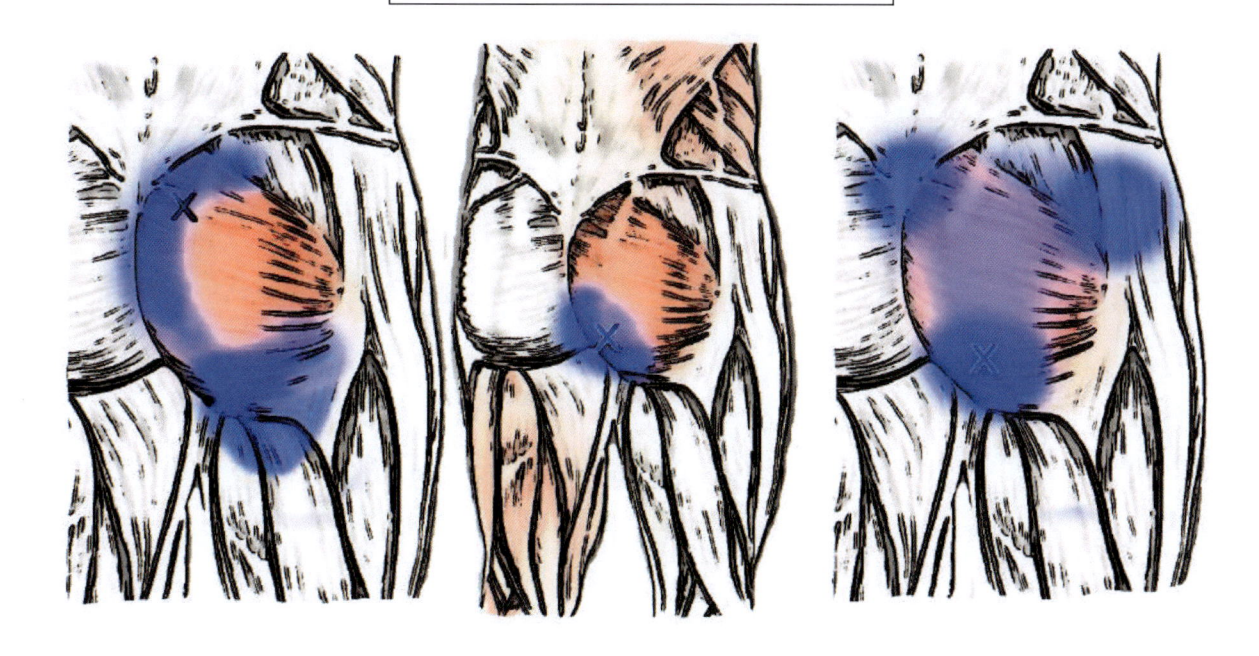

ADDUCTOR BREVIS & LONGUS
REF NO: 10

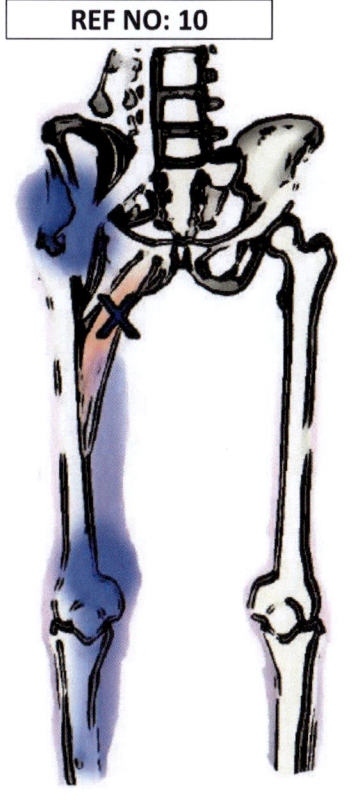

PSOAS & ILIACUS
REF NO: 11

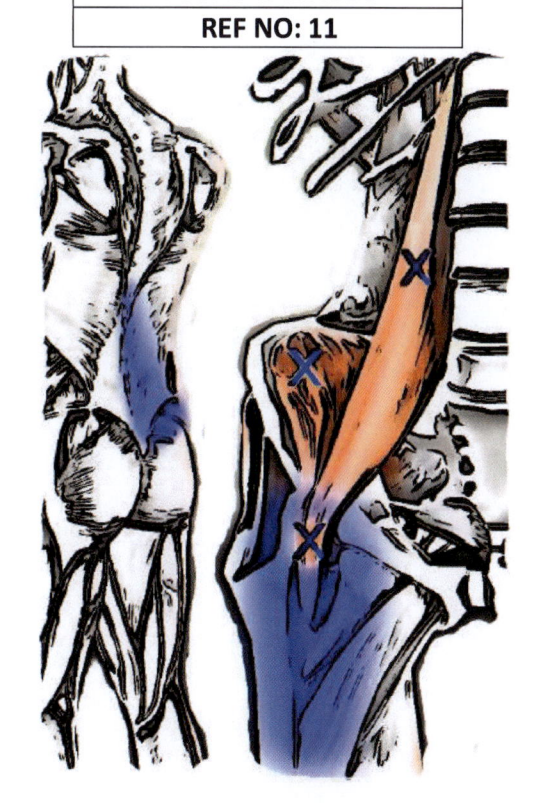

SARTORIUS
REF NO: 12

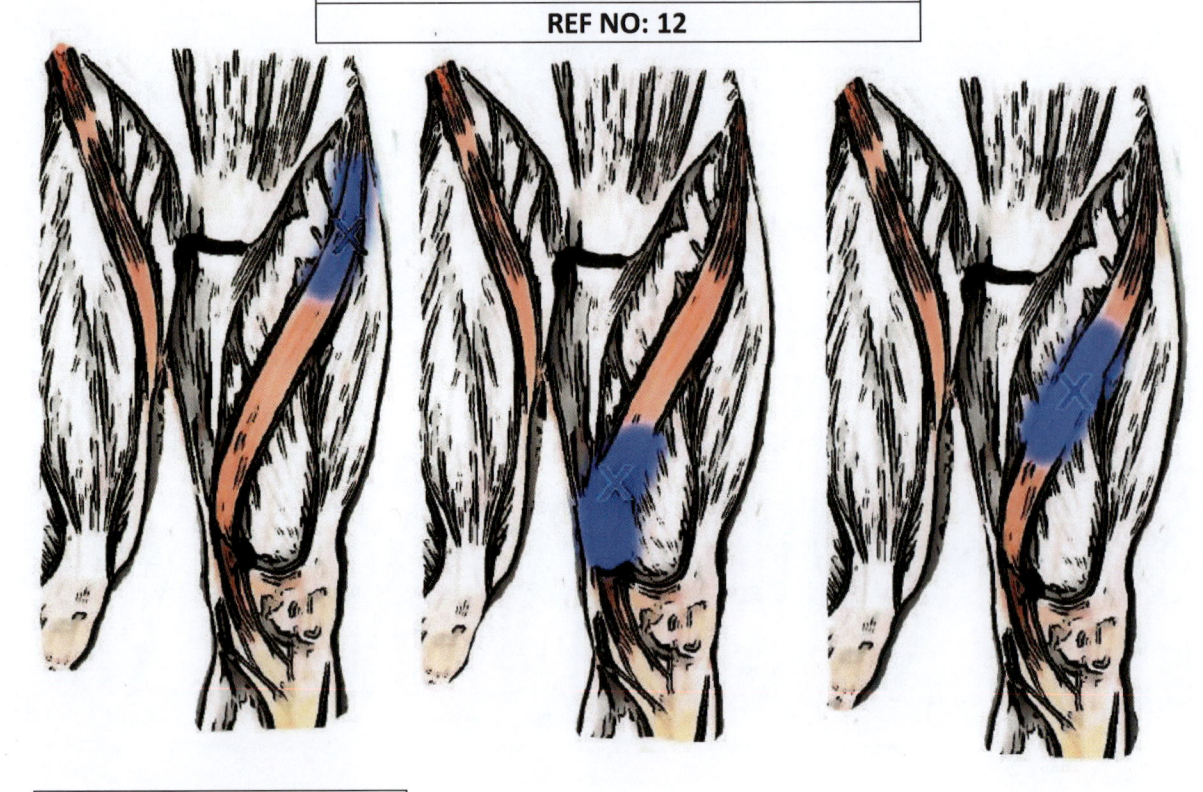

ADDUCTOR MAGNUS
REF NO: 14

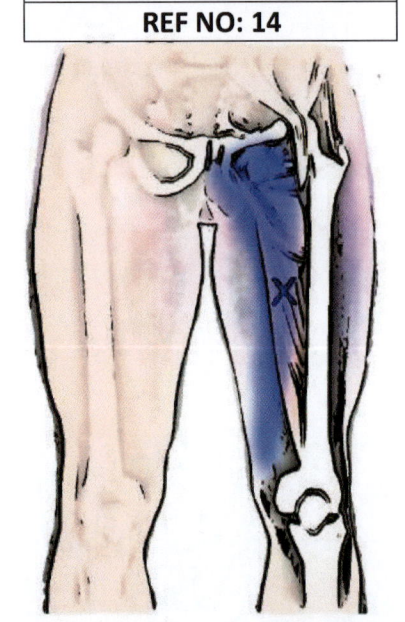

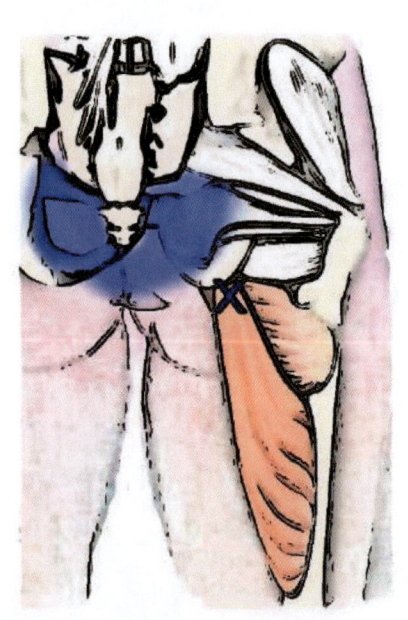

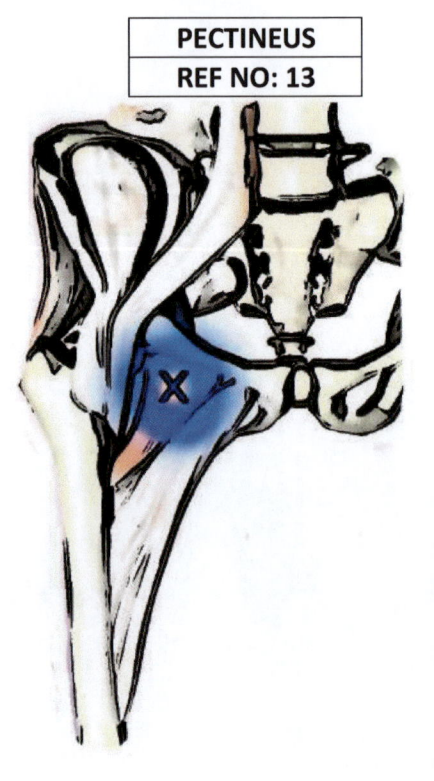

PECTINEUS
REF NO: 13

VASTUS MEDIALIS
REF NO: 15

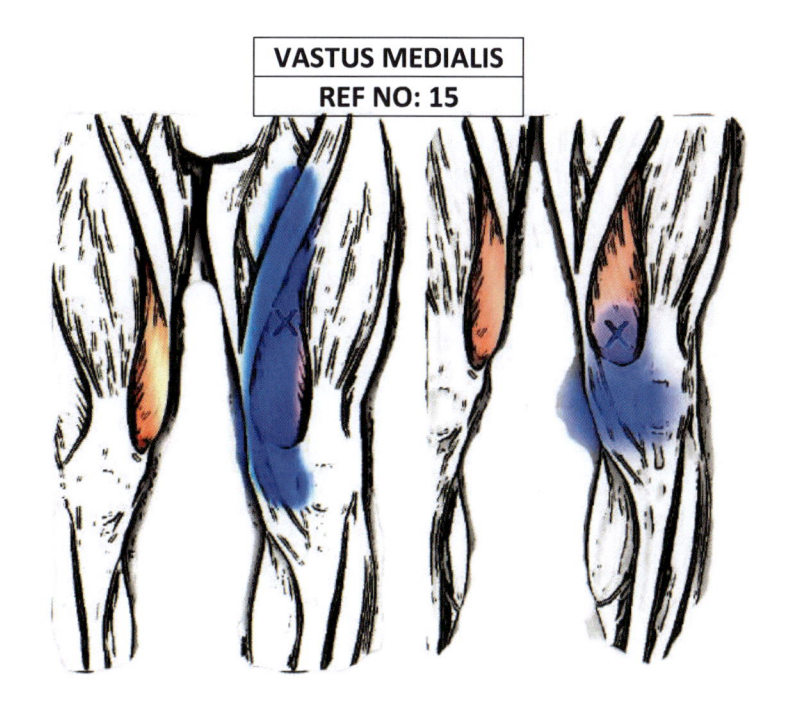

GRACILIS
REF NO: 16

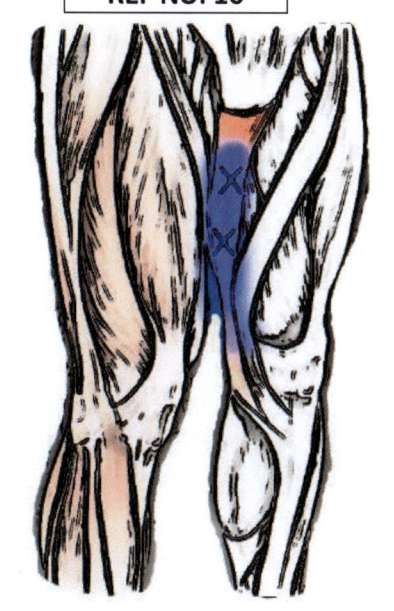

SEMITENDINOSUS & SEMIMEMBRANOSUS
REF NO: 17

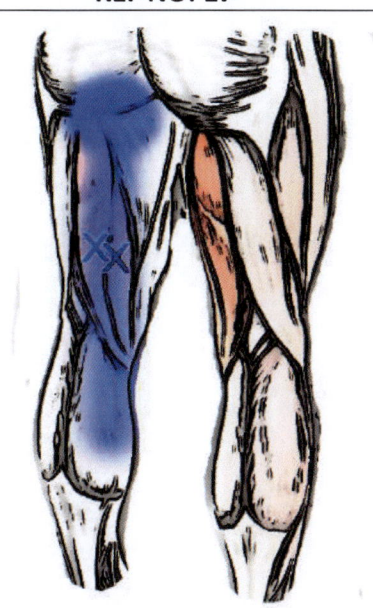

BICEPS FEMORIS
REF NO: 18

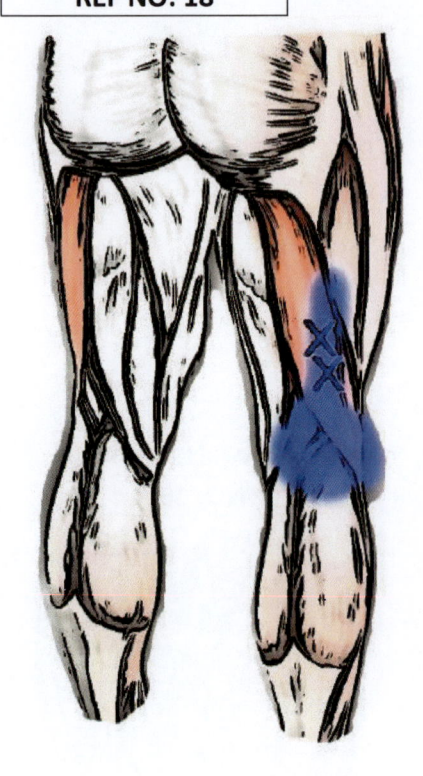

OBTURATOR INTERNUS
REF NO: 19

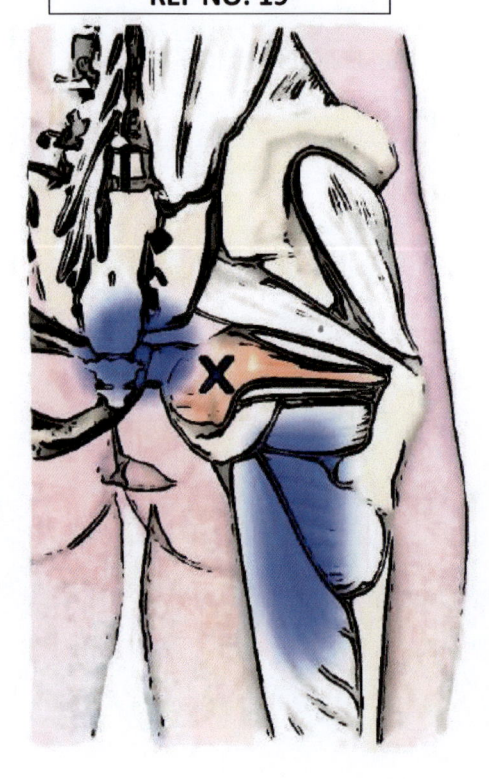

BUTTOCKS PAIN REFERRAL PAIN CHART/ DIAGRAMS

Location of Pain	Muscle	Referral	Picture Ref no:
Buttock Pain, Sacral Pain	Gluteus Medius	Trigger points near the sacrum refer pain into the sacrum. Trigger points in the middle aspect of the muscle refer down into the lateral hip with spillover into the thigh. The least common trigger points in the anterior portion refer along the Iliac Crest and back into the sacrum	Ref no: 1
Buttock Pain, Sacral Pain	Quadratus Lumborum	The uppermost trigger points refer pain to the SI joint and the lateral hip. The most inferior points refer to the buttock. The middle trigger point refer over the SI joint. Some people report a jolting pain to the anterior thigh from deep QL trigger points.	Ref no: 2
Buttock Pain, Sacral Pain	Gluteus Maximus	The trigger points near the sacrum refer pain in a crescent pattern from the sacrum down to the gluteal fold. The most common trigger point location is at the distal portion of the muscle, and refers to the entire buttock, and also deep into the buttock, which can lead to the false conclusion that deeper muscles are involved. The third trigger point lies on the most medial and inferior fibers, next to the coccyx.	Ref no: 3
Buttock Pain	Iliocostalis	Trigger points around T6 refer into the inferior portion of the scapula, and also into the chest area, which can mimic angina. Trigger points around T11 refer into the mid back with spillover upwards into the scapula and down into the ilium. This point can also refer into the abdominal region mimicking Visceral pain. The trigger point around L1 refers deep into the mid buttock	Ref no: 4
Buttock Pain	Longissimus	Primary referrals are downward. The referral pattern for the point around T11 is into the posterior hip, with spillover down the lower back. This point around L1 refers into the SI joint and Ilium. Both these points are common causes of lower back pain.	Ref no: 5

Buttock Pain	Semitendinosus and Semimembranosus	The main referral is up into the Gluteal fold, with spillover all along the posterior leg.	Ref no: 6
Buttock Pain	Piriformis	Trigger points refer pain into the sacro-iliac region, across the posterior hip, and down the thigh	Ref no: 7
Buttock Pain	Gluteus Minimus	Trigger points in the Anterior portion of this muscle refer down the lateral leg and into the buttock. Trigger points in the Posterior part of this muscle have a similar but more posterior referral pattern that does not go as far down the leg. Since the referral pattern of this muscle mimics Sciatica, this muscle should be first to be checked for involvement if the straight leg test turns out negative.	Ref no: 8
Buttock Pain, Sacral Pain	Rectus Abdominis	The upper trigger points rear to the mid-back, the lower points to the lower back. If you work on the back erector group is not providing relief, look to this muscle. The Rectus Abdominis will also be tight in clients that slouch, and have a posteriorly rotated pelvis.	Ref no: 9
Buttock Pain	Soleus	Distal trigger points refer down into the posterior and plantar surface of the ankle. Proximal trigger points refer into the posterior calf. The rarest trigger point in the distal lateral part of the muscle may refer pain into the sacrum.	Ref no: 10
Sacral Pain	Multifidi	Trigger points in the thoracic and lumbar sections refer around themselves. Trigger points at L2 and S1 also refer into the abdomen. Trigger points in the cervical region refer down into the scapula and posterior neck	Ref no: 11

BUTTOCKS PAIN CHART DIAGRAM

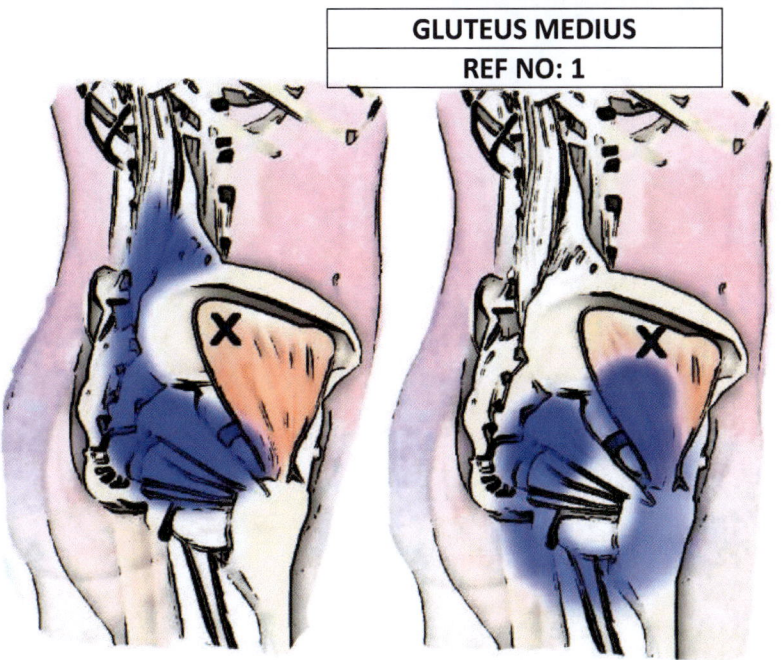

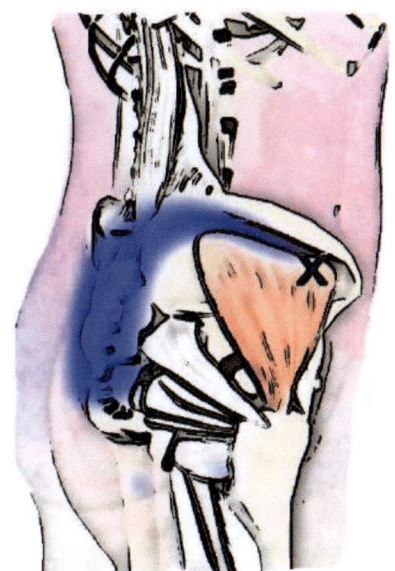

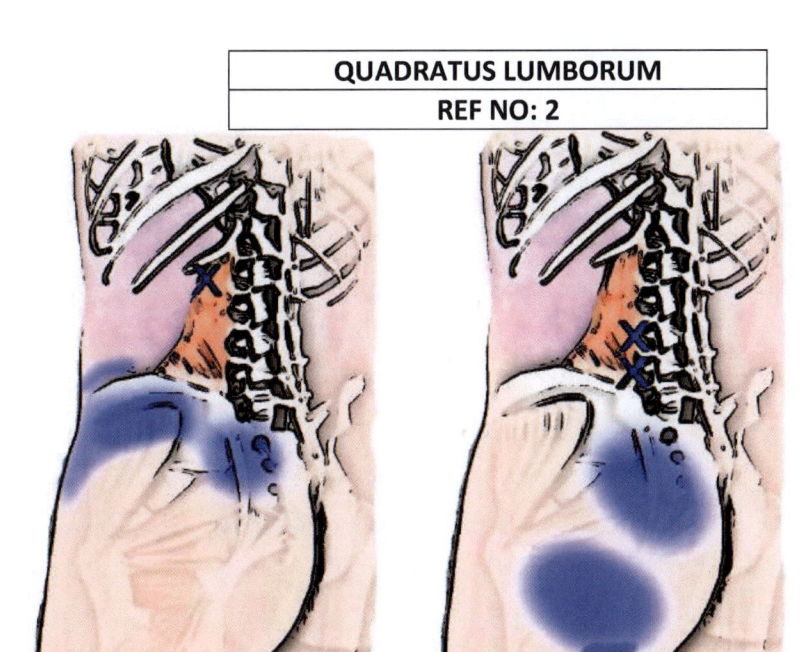

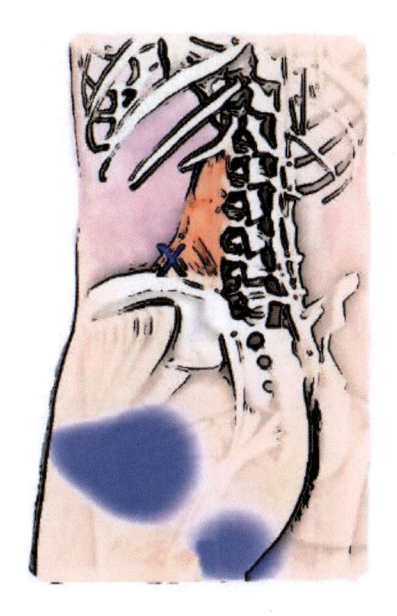

GLUTEUS MEDIUS
REF NO: 1

QUADRATUS LUMBORUM
REF NO: 2

GLUTEUS MAX
REF NO: 3

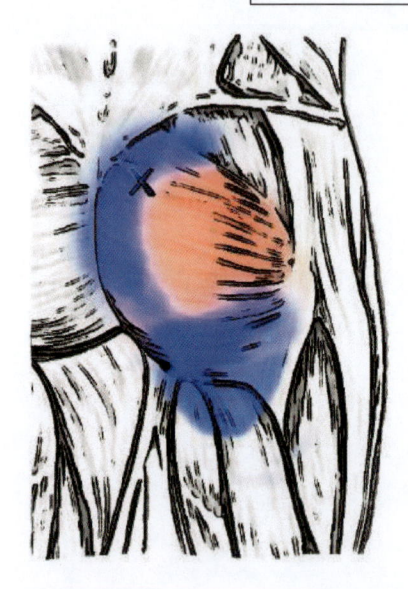

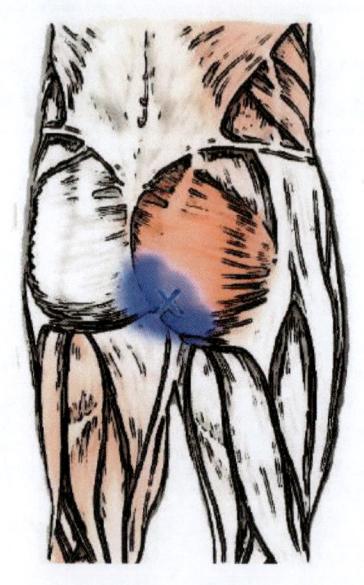

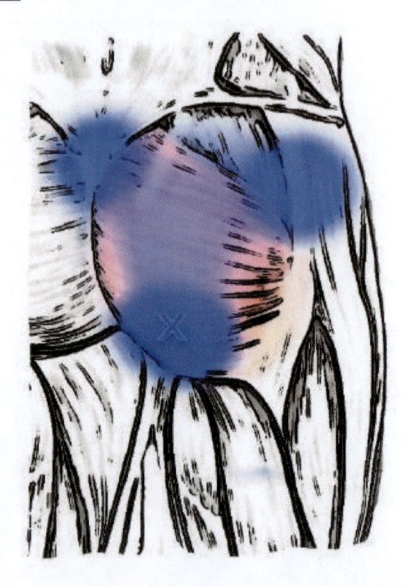

ILIOCOSTALIS
REF NO: 4

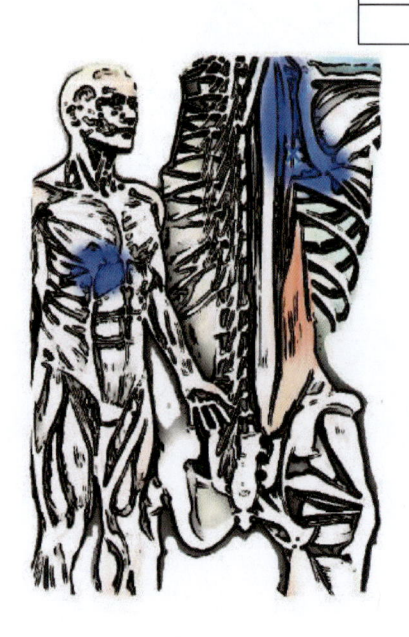

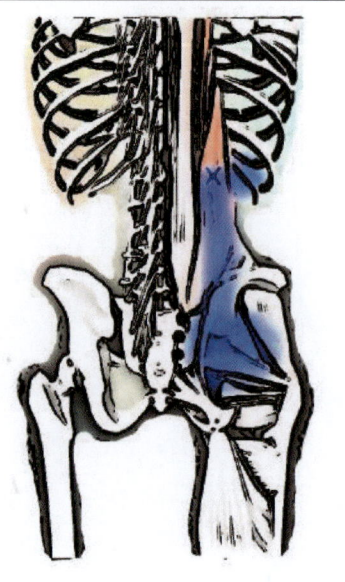

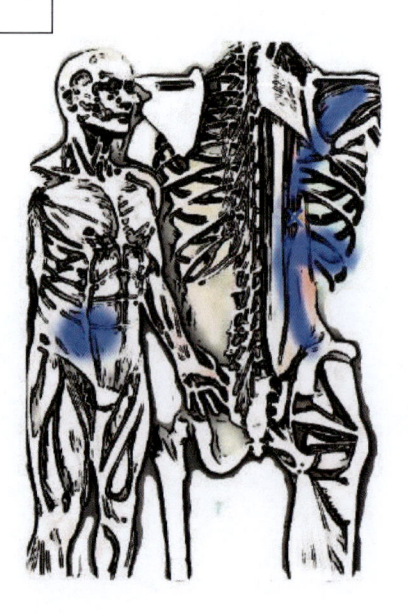

LONGISSIMUS
REF NO: 5

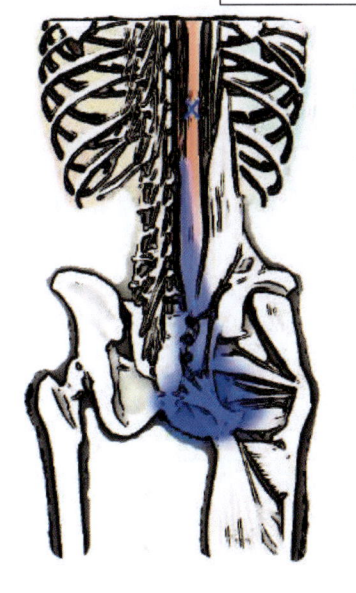

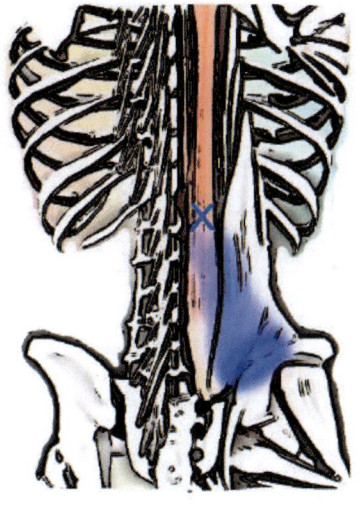

SEMITENDINOSUS & SEMIMEMBRANOSUS
REF NO: 6

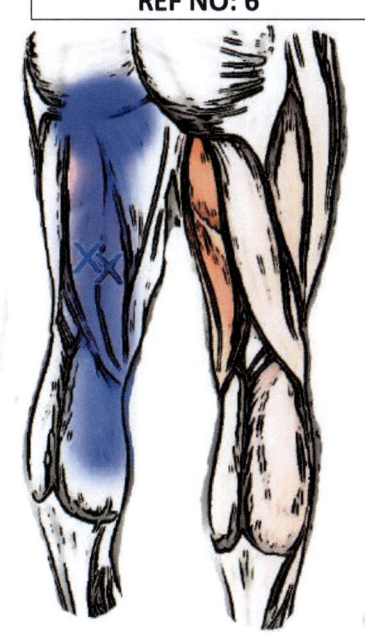

PIRIFORMIS
REF NO: 7

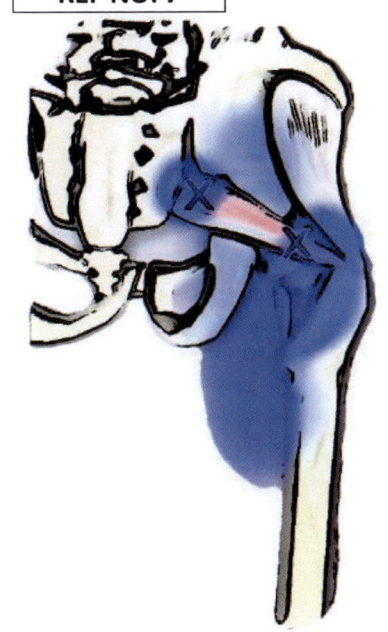

GLUTEUS MINIMUS
REF NO: 8

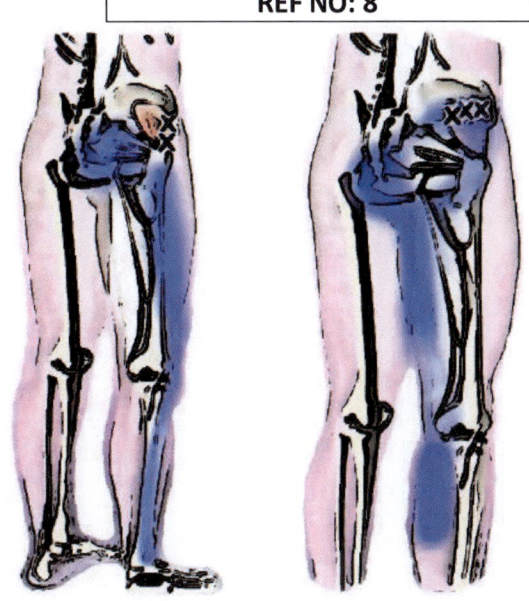

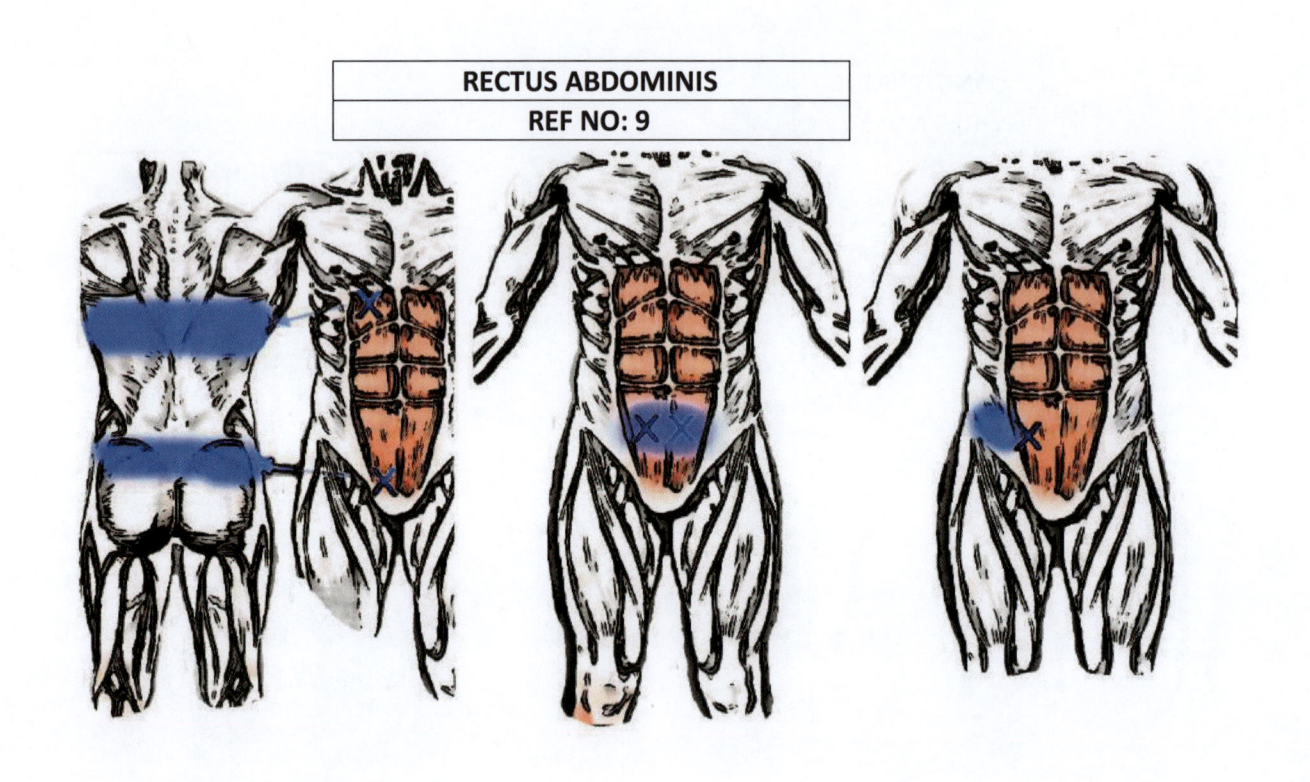

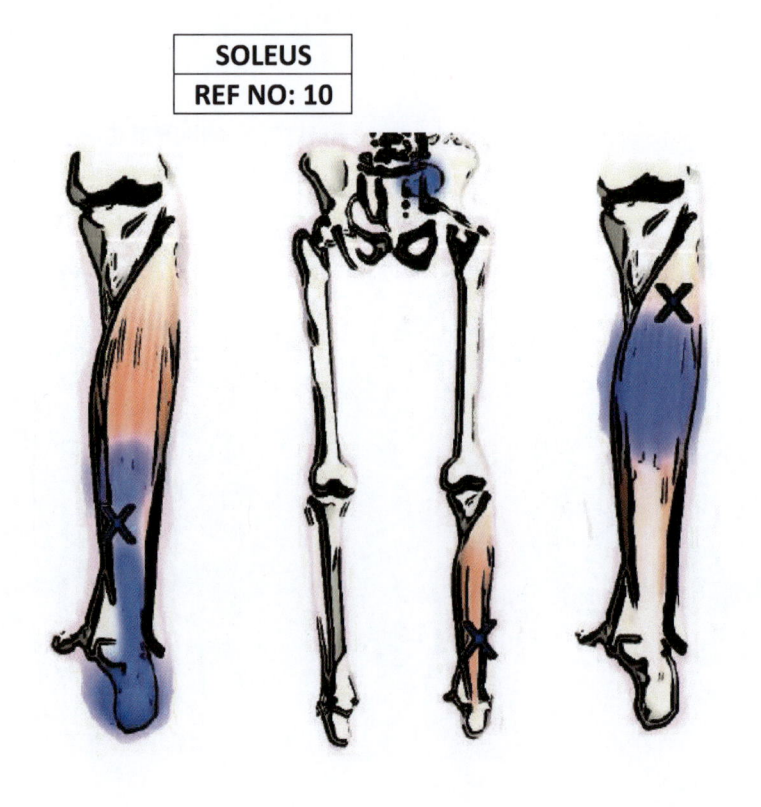

RECTUS ABDOMINIS
REF NO: 9

SOLEUS
REF NO: 10

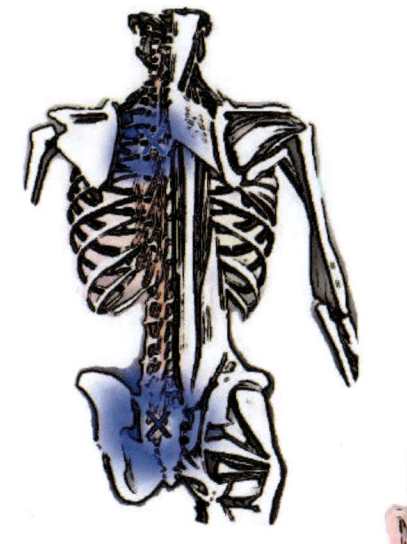

MULTIFIDI
REF NO: 11

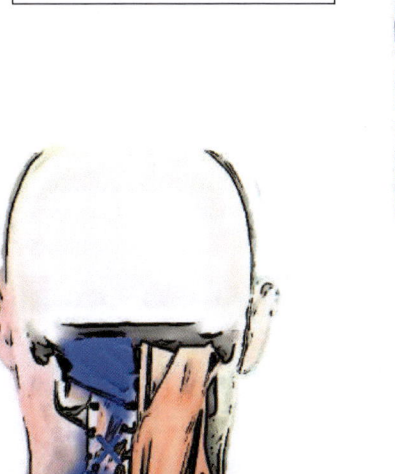

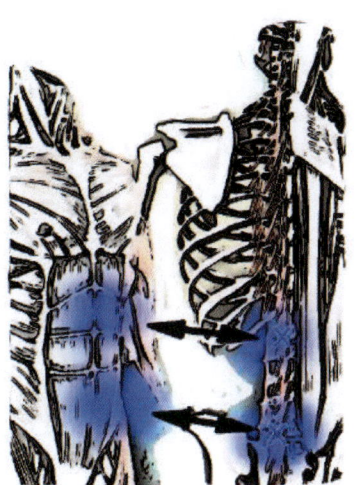

ABDOMINAL PAIN REFERRAL CHART / DIAGRAMS

Location of Pain	Muscle	Referral	Picture Ref no:
Abdominal Pain	Rectus Abdominis	The upper trigger points rear to the mid-back, the lower points to the lower back. If you work on the back erector group is not providing relief, look to this muscle. The Rectus Abdominis will also be tight in clients that slouch, and have a posteriorly rotated pelvis.	Ref no: 1
Abdominal Pain	External Obliques	Multiple referral patterns that run along the abdomen. Upper trigger points can mimic heart burn. Lower trigger points can refer into the inguinal ligament and genitals.	Ref no: 2
Abdominal Pain	Iliocostalis	Trigger points around T6 refer into the inferior portion of the scapula, and also into the chest area, which can mimic angina. Trigger points around T11 refer into the mid back with spillover upwards into the scapula and down into the ilium. This point can also refer into the abdominal region mimicking Visceral pain. The trigger point around L1 refers deep into the mid buttock	Ref no: 3
Abdominal Pain	Multifidi	Trigger points in the thoracic and lumbar sections refer around themselves. Trigger points at L2 and S1 also refer into the abdomen. Trigger points in the cervical region refer down into the scapula and posterior neck.	Ref no: 4

ABDOMINAL PAIN CHART DIAGRAMS

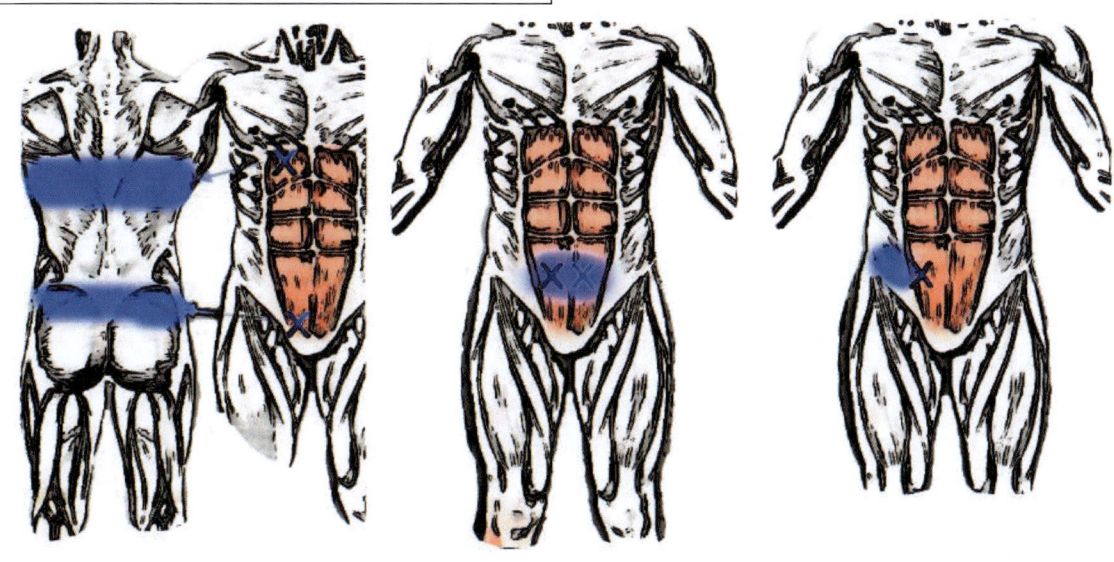

RECTUS ABDOMINIS
REF NO: 1

EXTERNAL OBLIQUES
REF NO: 2

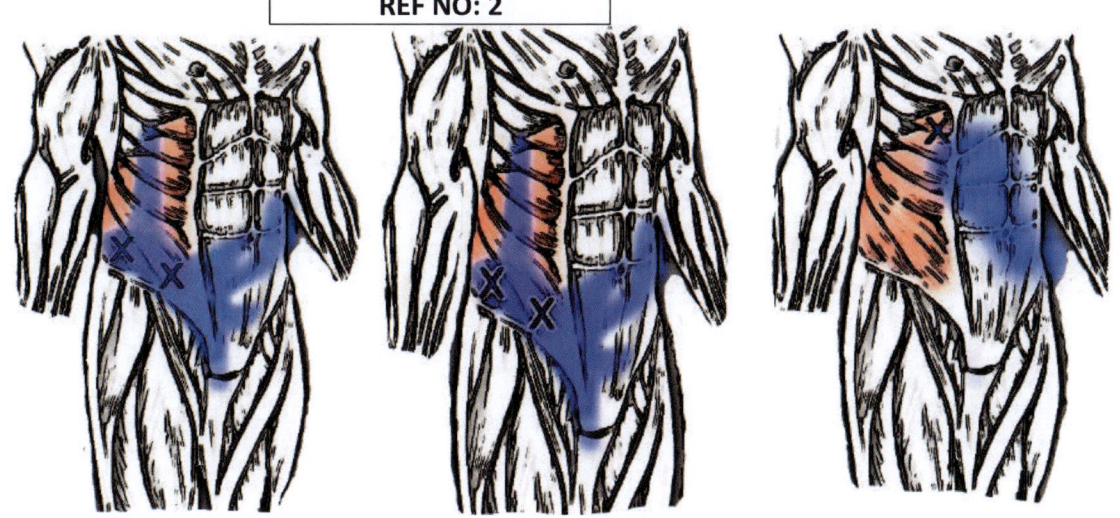

ILIOCOSTALIS
REF NO: 3

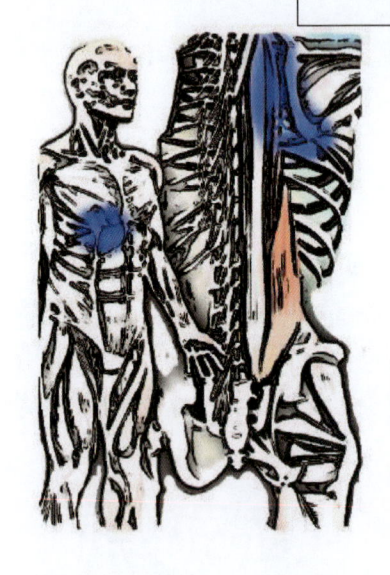

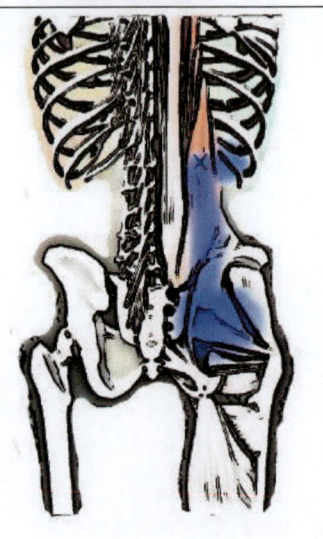

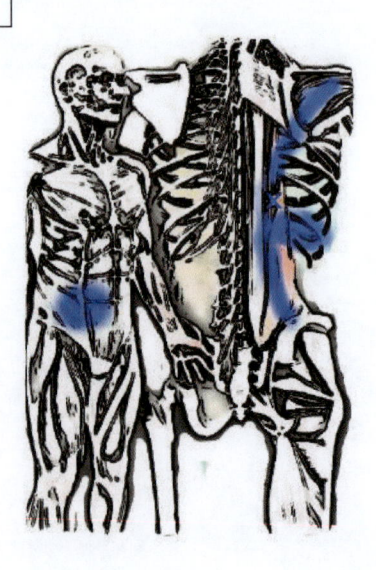

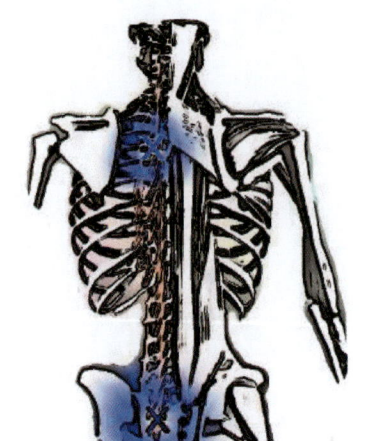

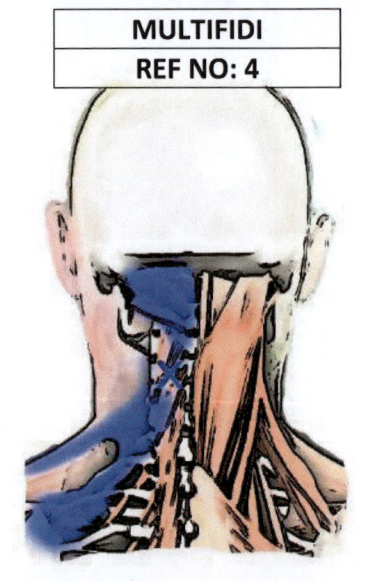

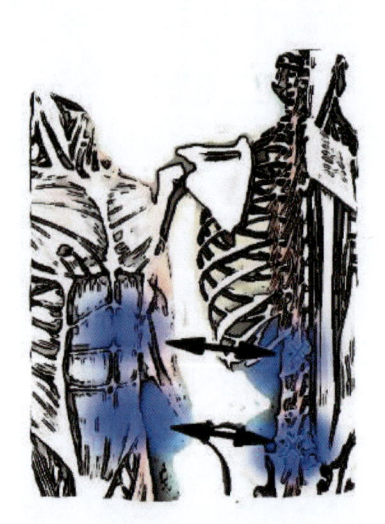

MULTIFIDI
REF NO: 4

BACK PAIN REFERRAL PAIN CHART / DIAGRAMS

Location of Pain	Muscle	Referral	Picture Ref no:
Lower Back Pain	Gluteus Medius	Trigger points near the sacrum refer pain into the sacrum. Trigger points in the middle aspect of the muscle refer down into the lateral hip with spillover into the thigh. The least common trigger points in the anterior portion refer along the Iliac Crest and back into the sacrum	Ref no: 1
Lower Back Pain	Multifidi	Trigger points in the thoracic and lumbar sections refer around themselves. Trigger points at L2 and S1 also refer into the abdomen. Trigger points in the cervical region refer down into the scapula and posterior neck.	Ref no: 2
Lower Back Pain	Psoas and Iliacus	Primarily to the lower lumbar area and sacrum, and secondly to the anterior thigh	Ref no: 3
Lower Back Pain	Longissimus	Primary referrals are downward. The referral pattern for the point around T11 is into the posterior hip, with spillover down into the lower back. This point around L1 refers into the SI joint and Ilium. Both these points are common causes of lower back pain.	Ref no: 4
Lower Back Pain	Rectus Abdominis	The upper trigger points rear to the mid-back, the lower points to the lower back. If you work on the back erector group is not providing relief, look to this muscle. The Rectus Abdominis will also be tight in clients that slouch, and have a posteriorly rotated pelvis.	Ref no: 5
Lower Back Pain	Iliocostalis	Trigger points around T6 refer into the inferior portion of the scapula, and also into the chest area, which can mimic angina. Trigger points around T11 refer into the mid back with spillover upwards into the scapula and down into the ilium. This point can also refer into the abdominal region mimicking Visceral pain. The trigger point around L1 refers deep into the mid buttock	Ref no: 6

Upper Back Pain	Scalene Muscles	Trigger points in these muscles can refer in two finger-like projections into the chest. Other common patterns are into the shoulder, scapula and down the lateral arm, into the thumb and index finger. The Scalenes can impinge on the Brachial Plexus, causing nerve pain or numbness down the arm. This is called Thoracic Outlet Syndrome.	Ref no: 7
Upper Back Pain	Levator Scapula	Refers to the angle of the neck with spillover into the scapula. To help this muscle, you must get the head back by releasing the anterior chest and neck musculature.	Ref no: 8
Upper Back Pain	Trapezius	Trigger points on the lateral upper edge refer into lateral neck and temples, causing "tension neck ache". Other points in the middle and lower fibers refer into the posterior neck and shoulders.	Ref no: 9
Upper Back Pain	Multifidi	Trigger points in the thoracic and lumbar sections refer around themselves. Trigger points at L2 and S1 also refer into the abdomen. Trigger points in the cervical region refer down into the scapula and posterior neck.	Ref no: 10
Upper Back Pain	Rhomboids	Trigger points in the Rhomboids refer locally to the upper back.	Ref no: 11
Upper Back Pain	Splenius Cervicis	The lower trigger point refers pain into the angle of the neck. The upper point shoots pain from the inside of the head to the back of the eye.	Ref no: 12

BACK PAIN CHART DIAGRAMS

GLUTEUS MEDIUS
REF NO: 1

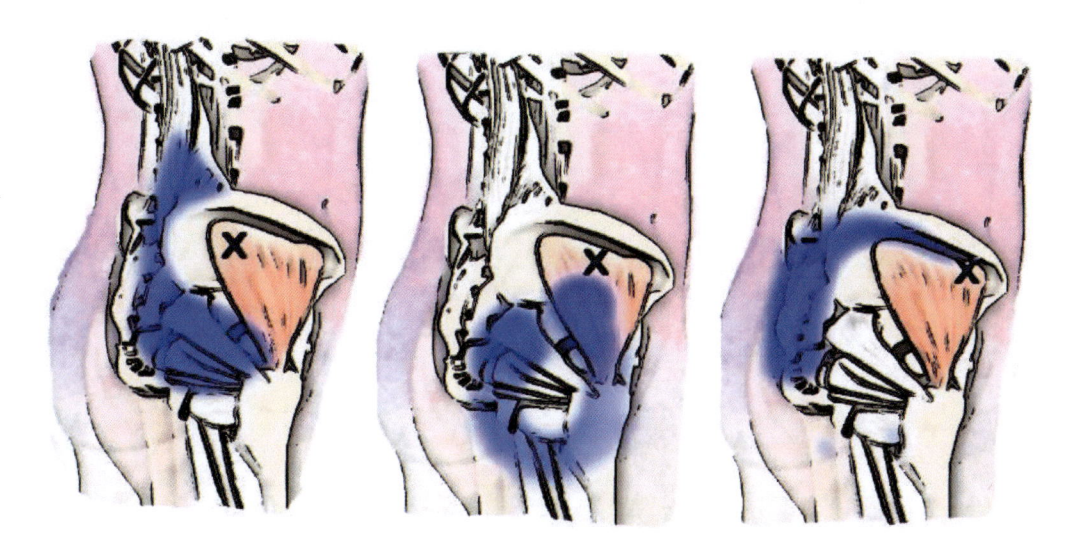

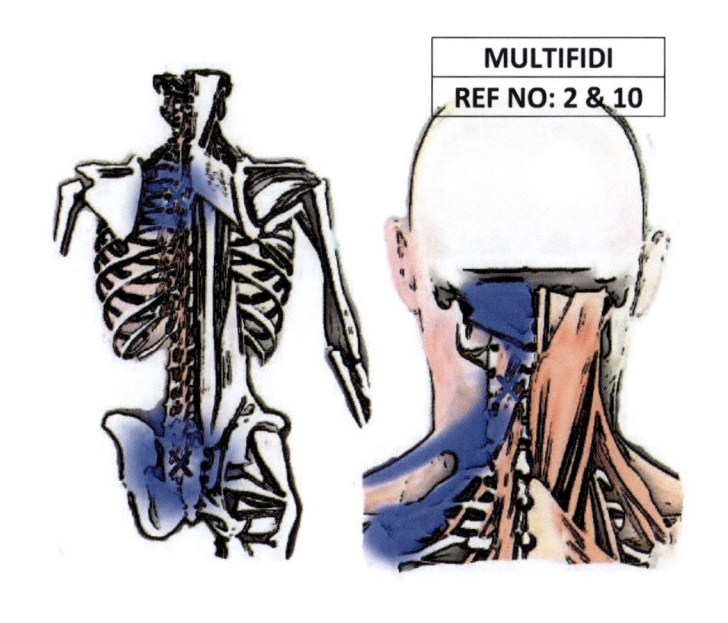

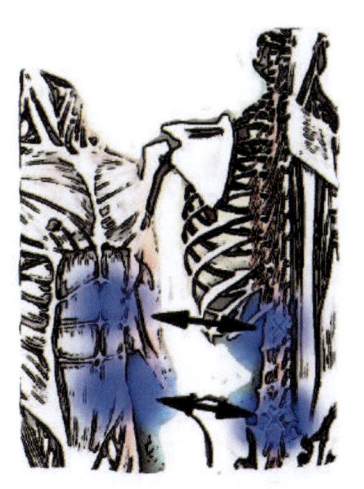

MULTIFIDI
REF NO: 2 & 10

PSOAS & ILIACUS
REF NO: 3

LONGISSIMUS
REF NO: 4

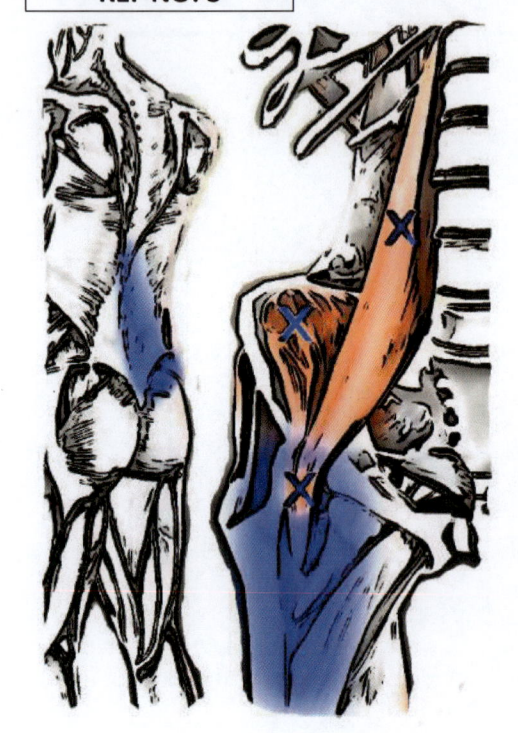

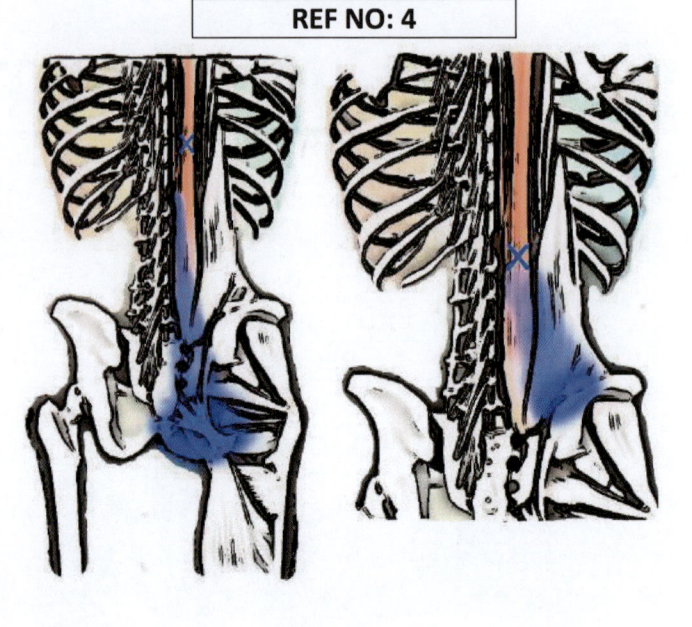

RECTUS ABDOMINIS
REF NO:5

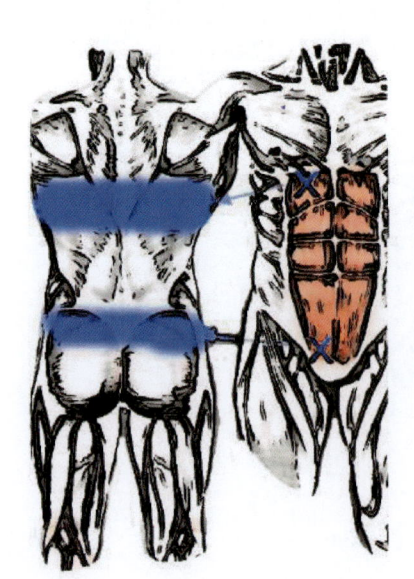

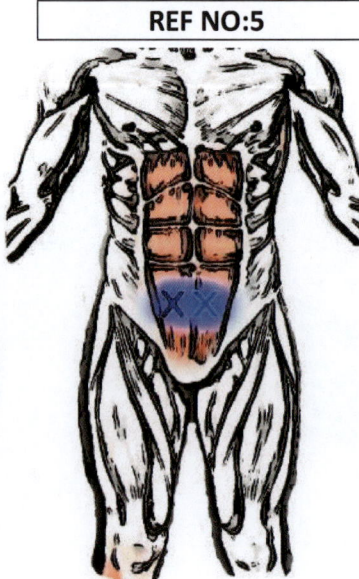

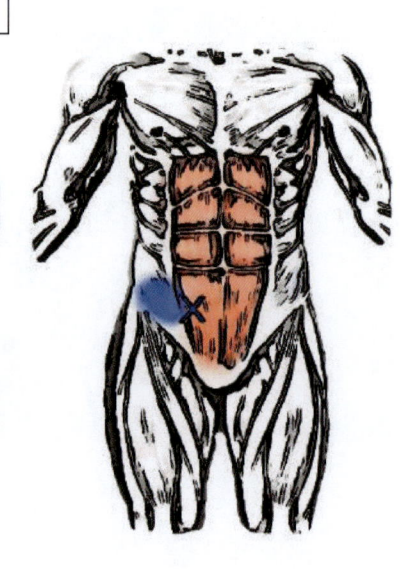

62

ILIOCOSTALIS
REF NO: 6

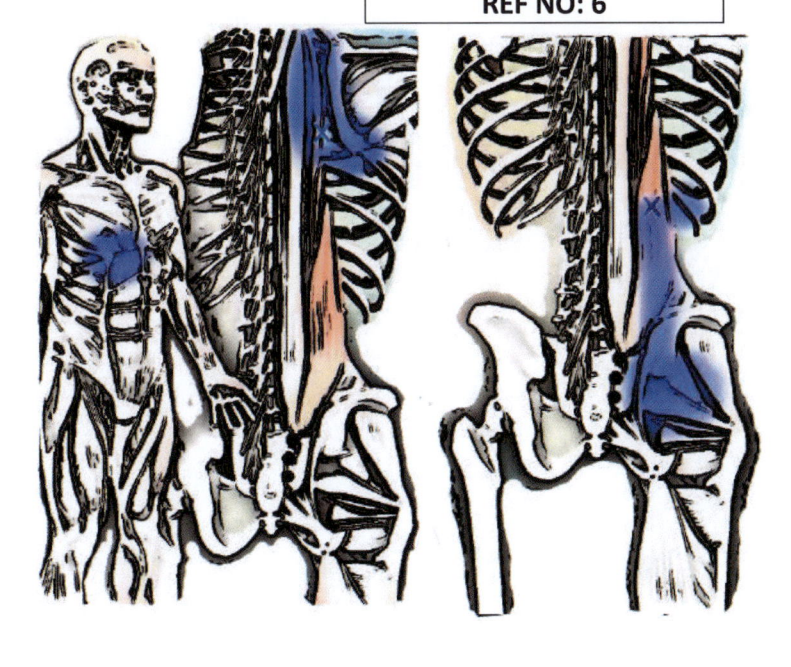

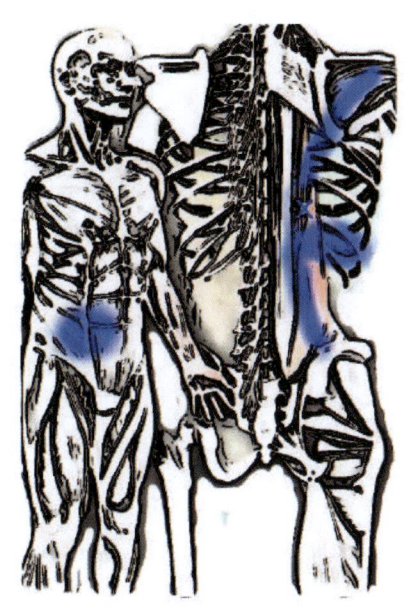

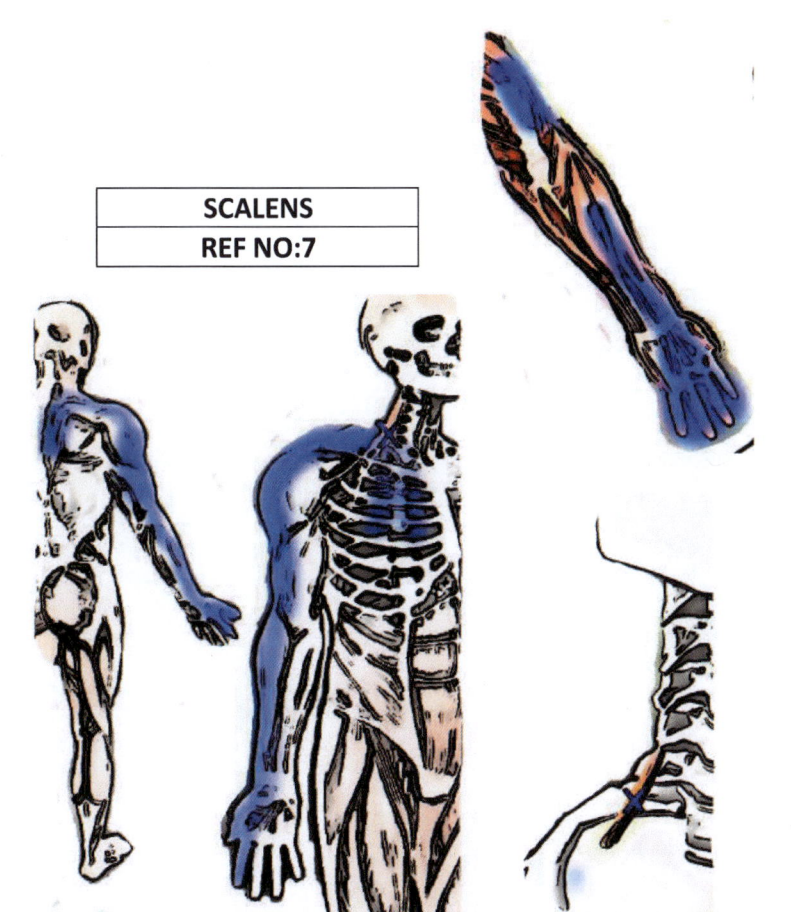

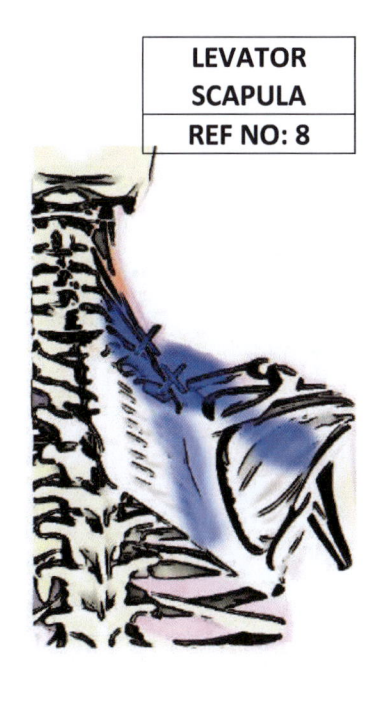

SCALENS
REF NO: 7

LEVATOR SCAPULA
REF NO: 8

63

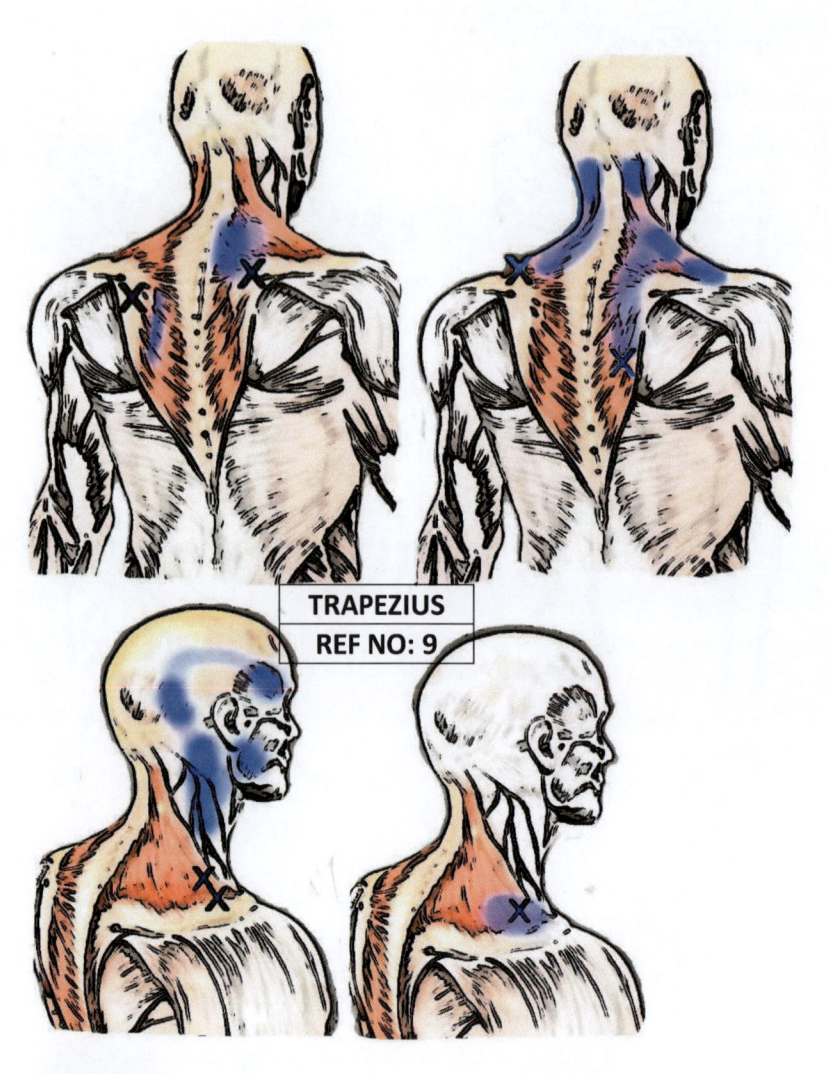

TRAPEZIUS
REF NO: 9

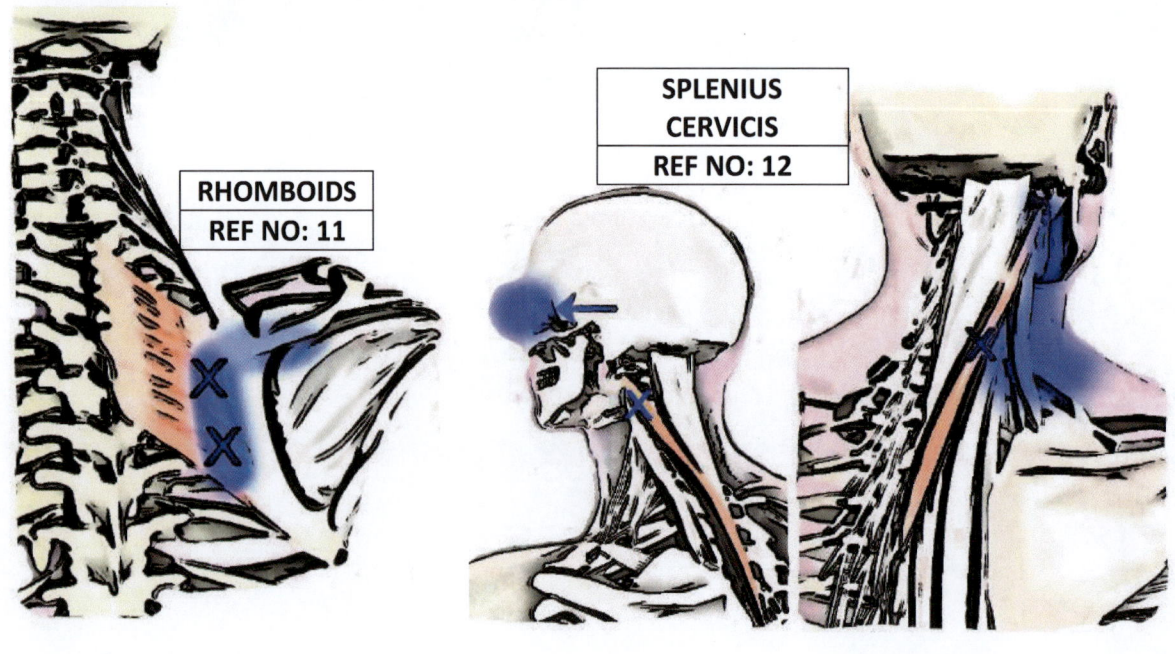

RHOMBOIDS
REF NO: 11

SPLENIUS CERVICIS
REF NO: 12

NECK AND SHOULDER PAIN REFERRAL CHART / DIAGRAMS

Location of Pain	Muscle	Referral	Picture Ref no:
Posterior Neck Pain	Trapezius	Trigger points on the lateral upper edge refer into lateral neck and temples, causing "tension neck ache". Other points in the middle and lower fibers refer into the posterior neck and shoulders.	Ref no: 1
Posterior Neck Pain	Multifidi	Trigger points in the thoracic and lumbar sections refer around themselves. Trigger points at L2 and S1 also refer into the abdomen. Trigger points in the cervical region refer down into the scapula and posterior neck.	Ref no: 2
Posterior Neck Pain	Levator Scapula	Referring to the angle of the neck with spillover into the scapula. To help this muscle, you must get the head back by releasing the anterior chest and neck musculature.	Ref no: 3
Posterior Neck Pain	Splenius Cervicis	The lower trigger point refers pain into the angle of the neck. The upper point shoots pain from the inside of the head to the back of the eye.	Ref no: 4
Posterior Neck Pain	Infraspinatus	The main referral pattern is deep into the anterior shoulder joint, with spillover down the anterior aspect of the arm. Less common trigger points near the lower medial border refer pain into the Rhomboids.	Ref no: 5
Posterior Shoulder Pain	Deltoid	Trigger points in the anterior Deltoid refer into the anterior and lateral shoulder. Trigger points in the posterior Deltoid refer into the posterior shoulder with spillover down the lateral arm.	Ref no: 6
Posterior Shoulder Pain	Levator Scapula	Refers to the angle of the neck with spillover into the scapula. To help this muscle, you must get the head back by releasing the anterior chest and neck musculature.	Ref no: 7
Posterior Shoulder Pain	Scalene Muscles	Trigger points in these muscles can refer in two finger-like projections into the chest. Other common patterns are into the shoulder, scapula and down the lateral arm, into the thumb and index finger. The Scalenes can impinge on the Brachial Plexus, causing nerve pain or numbness down the arm. This is called Thoracic Outlet Syndrome.	Ref no: 8

Posterior Shoulder Pain	Supraspinatus	The primary referral is a deep ache in the mid deltoid area, with spillover down the arm and into the elbow.	Ref no: 9
Posterior Shoulder Pain	Teres Major	Primary referral pattern is deep in the posterior deltoid region, with spillover infrequently into the dorsal part of the forearm.	Ref no: 10
Posterior Shoulder Pain	Teres Minor	Pain is referred into the posterior deltoid, and down the posterior arm.	Ref no: 11
Posterior Shoulder Pain	Subscapularis	The Subscapularis primarily refers to the posterior shoulder with spillover into the posterior medial aspect of the arm and both sides of the wrist.	Ref no: 12
Posterior Shoulder Pain	Latissimus Dorsi	The main trigger point location for this muscle refers pain into the inferior scapular area, with spillover down the posterior side of the arm and hand. An unusual trigger point in the anterior mid muscle refers pain inferiorly and sometimes into the anterior shoulder.	Ref no: 13
Posterior Shoulder Pain	Triceps	The long head usually refers pain into the posterior shoulder and sometimes down into the posterior forearm (skipping the elbow). Trigger points in the centre of the medial head refer into the Olecranon Process. The trigger points in the lateral part of the medial head refer to the lateral epicondyle, and are a common component of "Tennis Elbow".	Ref no: 14
Posterior Shoulder Pain	Trapezius	Trigger points on the lateral upper edge refer into lateral neck and temples, causing "tension neck ache". Other points in the middle and lower fibers refer into the posterior neck and shoulders.	Ref no: 15
Posterior Shoulder Pain	Iliocostalis	Trigger points around T6 refer into the inferior portion of the scapula, and also into the chest area, which can mimic angina. Trigger points around T11 refer into the mid back with spillover upwards into the scapula and down into the ilium. This point can also refer into the abdominal region mimicking Visceral pain. The trigger point around L1 refers deep into the mid buttock	Ref no: 16

NECK & SHOULDER PAIN CHART DIAGRAMS

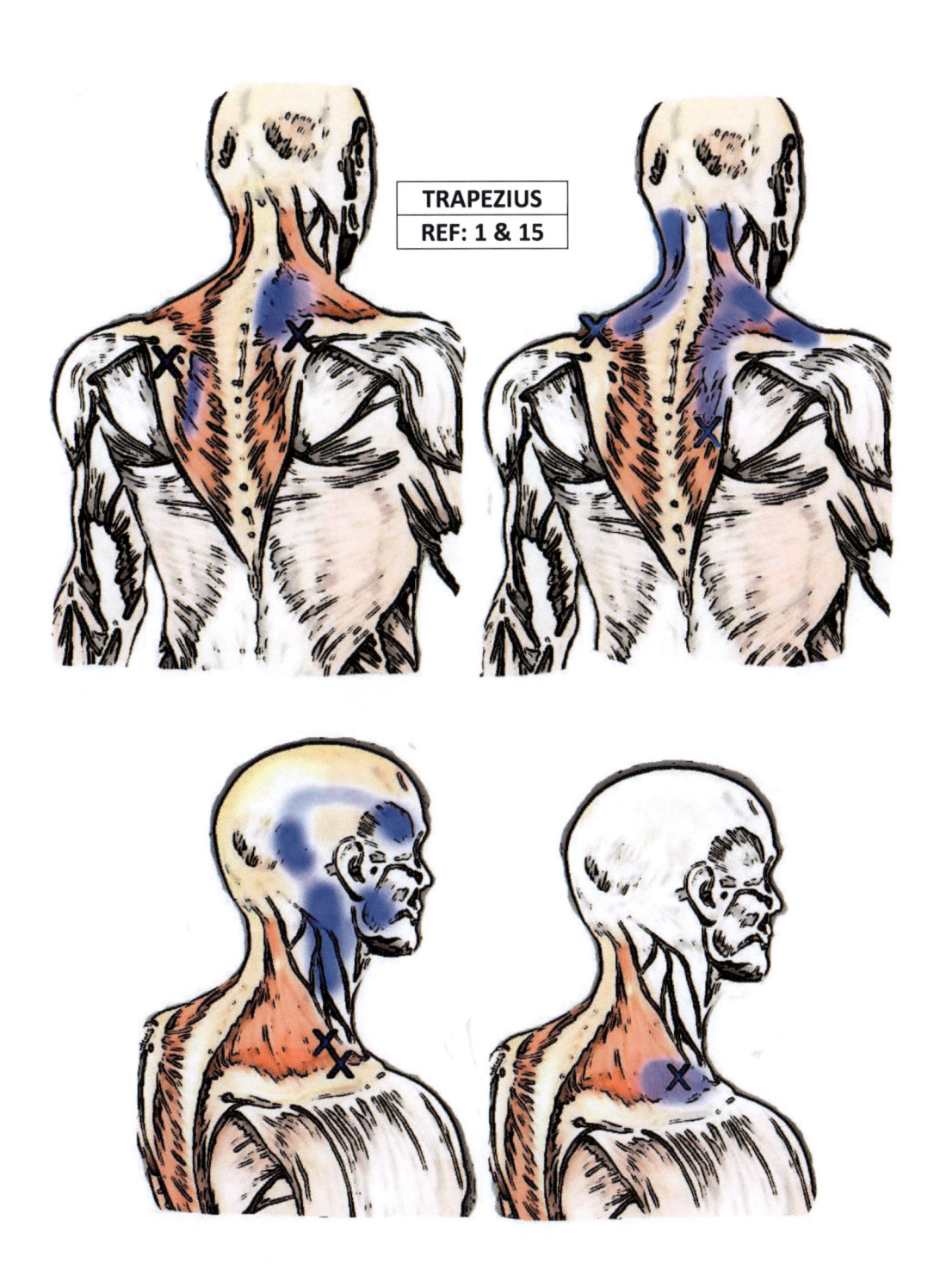

TRAPEZIUS
REF: 1 & 15

67

MULTIFIDI
REF NO: 2

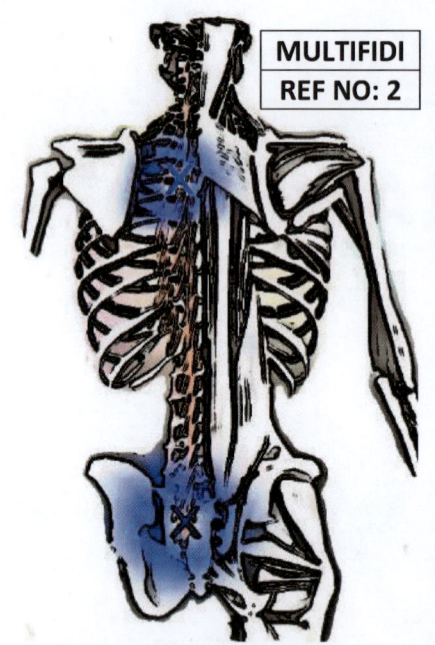

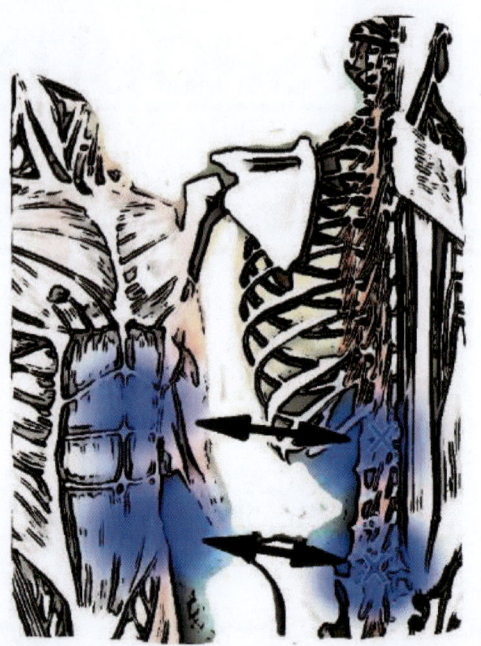

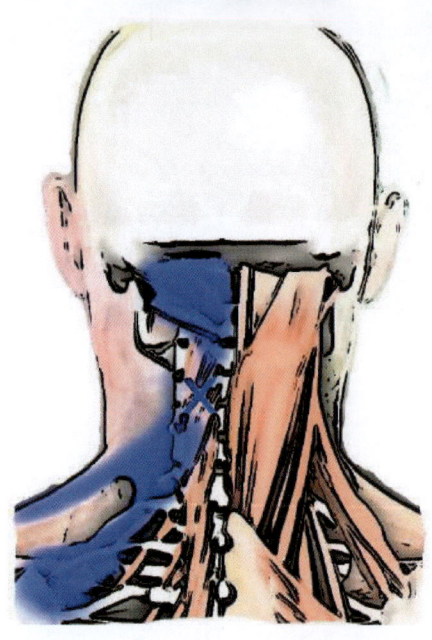

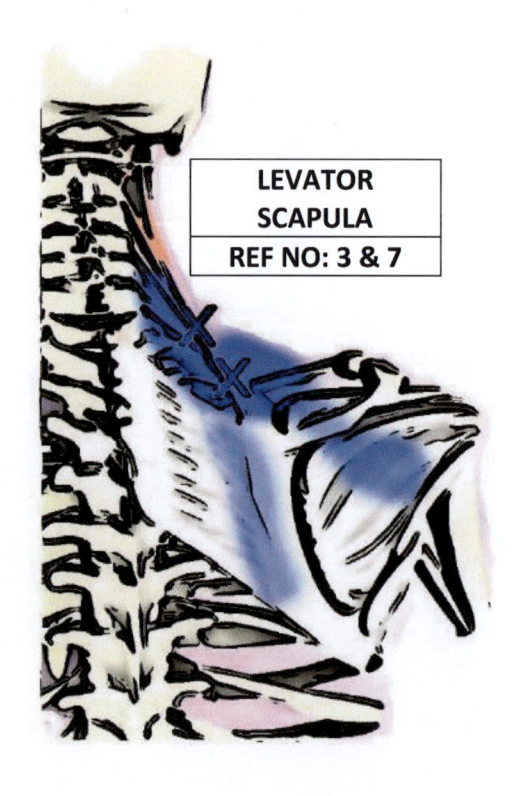

LEVATOR SCAPULA
REF NO: 3 & 7

SPLENIUS CERVICIS
REF NO: 4

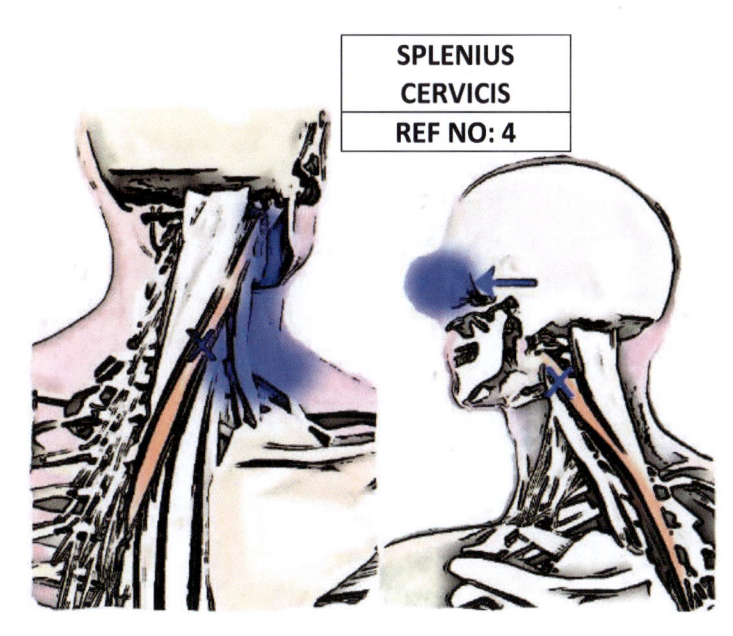

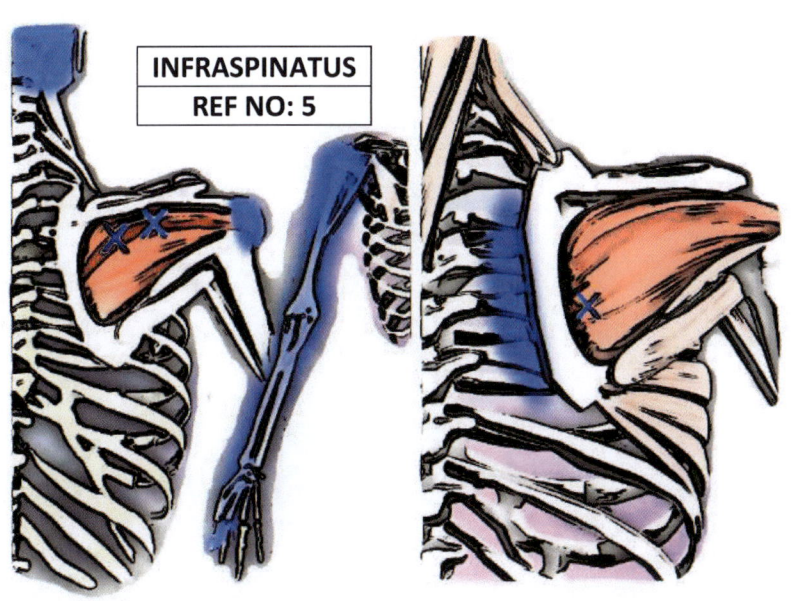

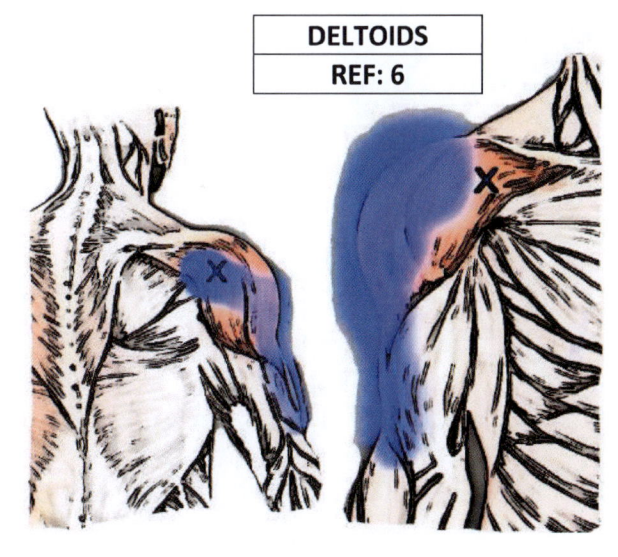

INFRASPINATUS
REF NO: 5

DELTOIDS
REF: 6

SUPRASPINATUS
REF NO: 9

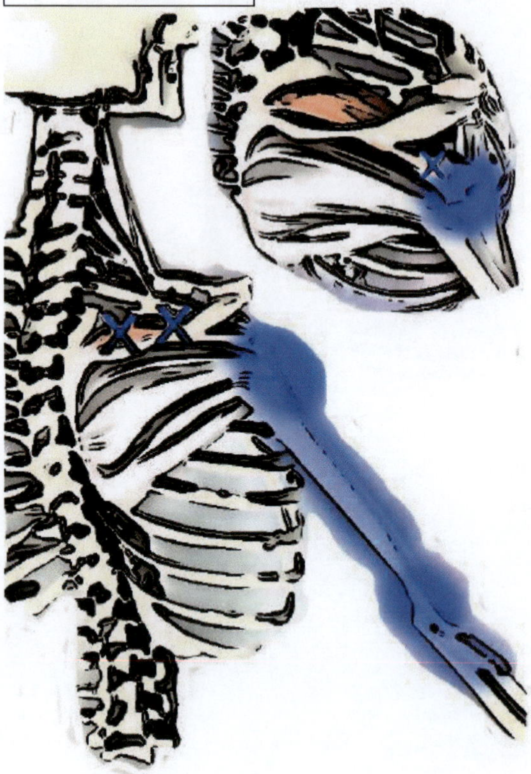

TERES MAJOR
REF NO: 10

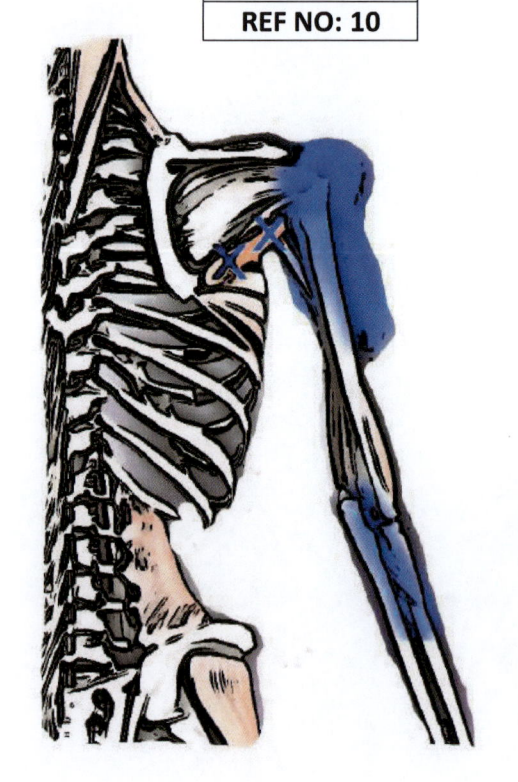

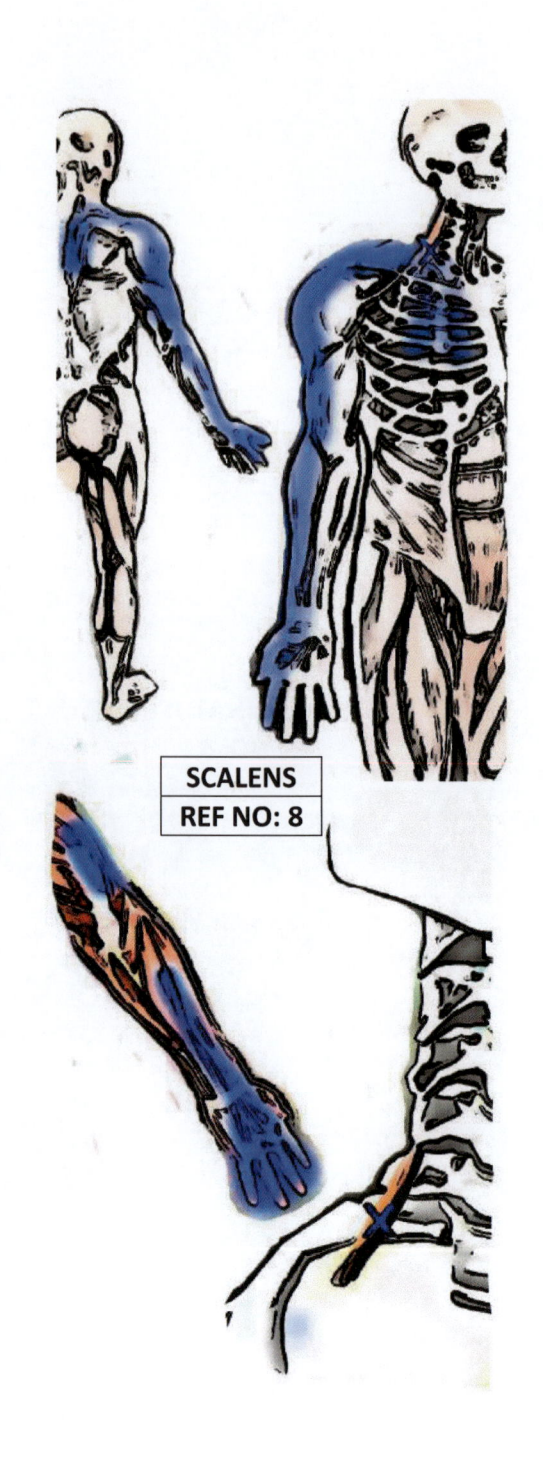

SCALENS
REF NO: 8

TERES MINOR
REF NO: 11

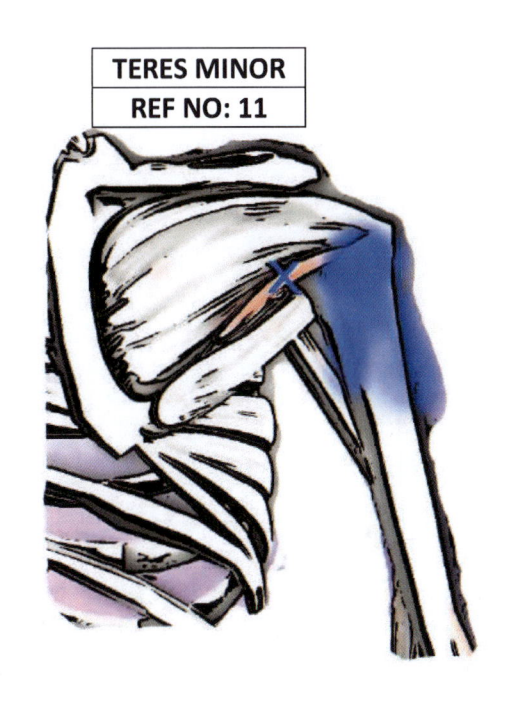

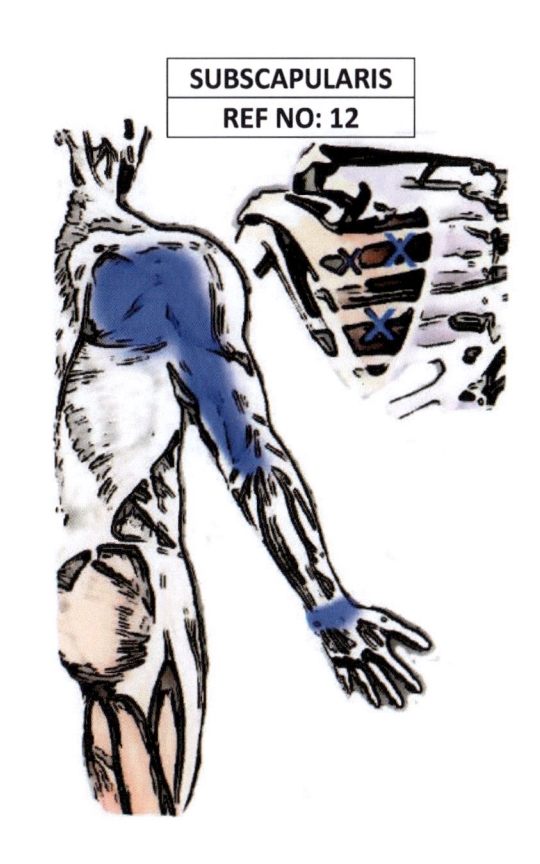

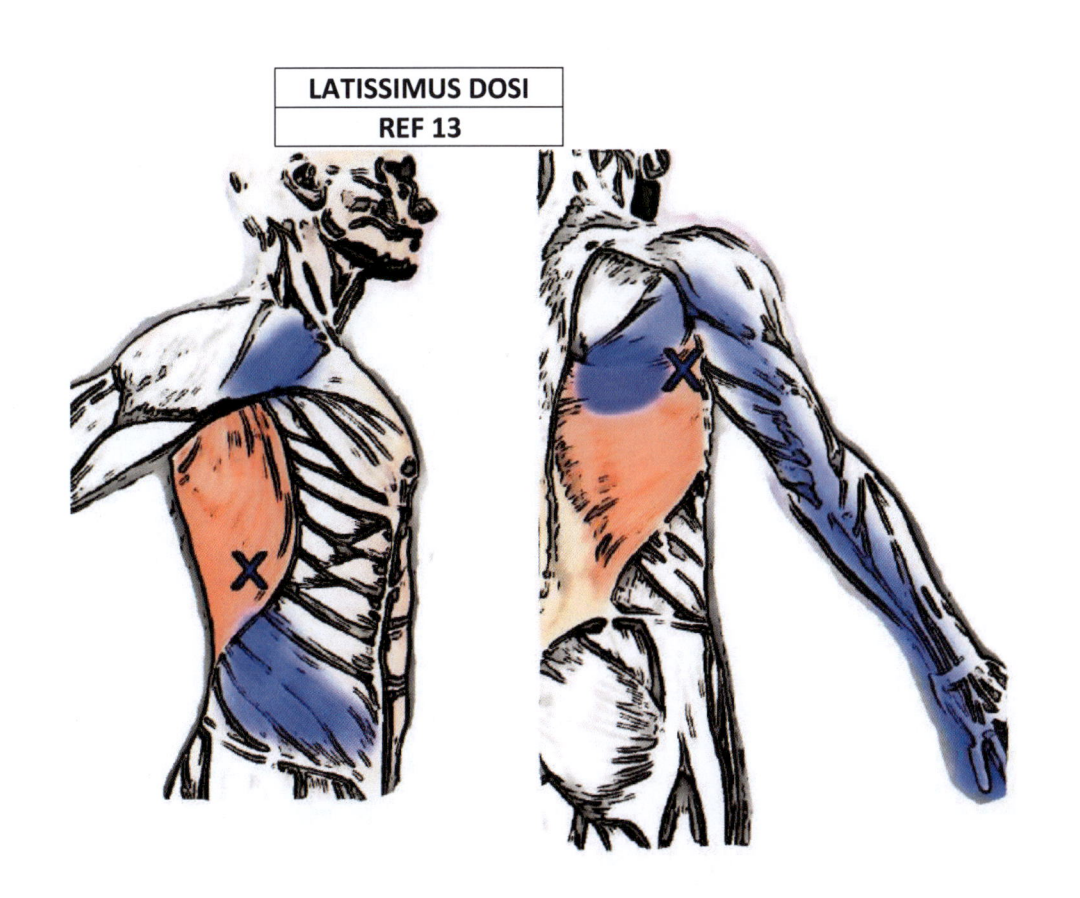

SUBSCAPULARIS
REF NO: 12

LATISSIMUS DOSI
REF 13

TRICEPS
REF NO: 14

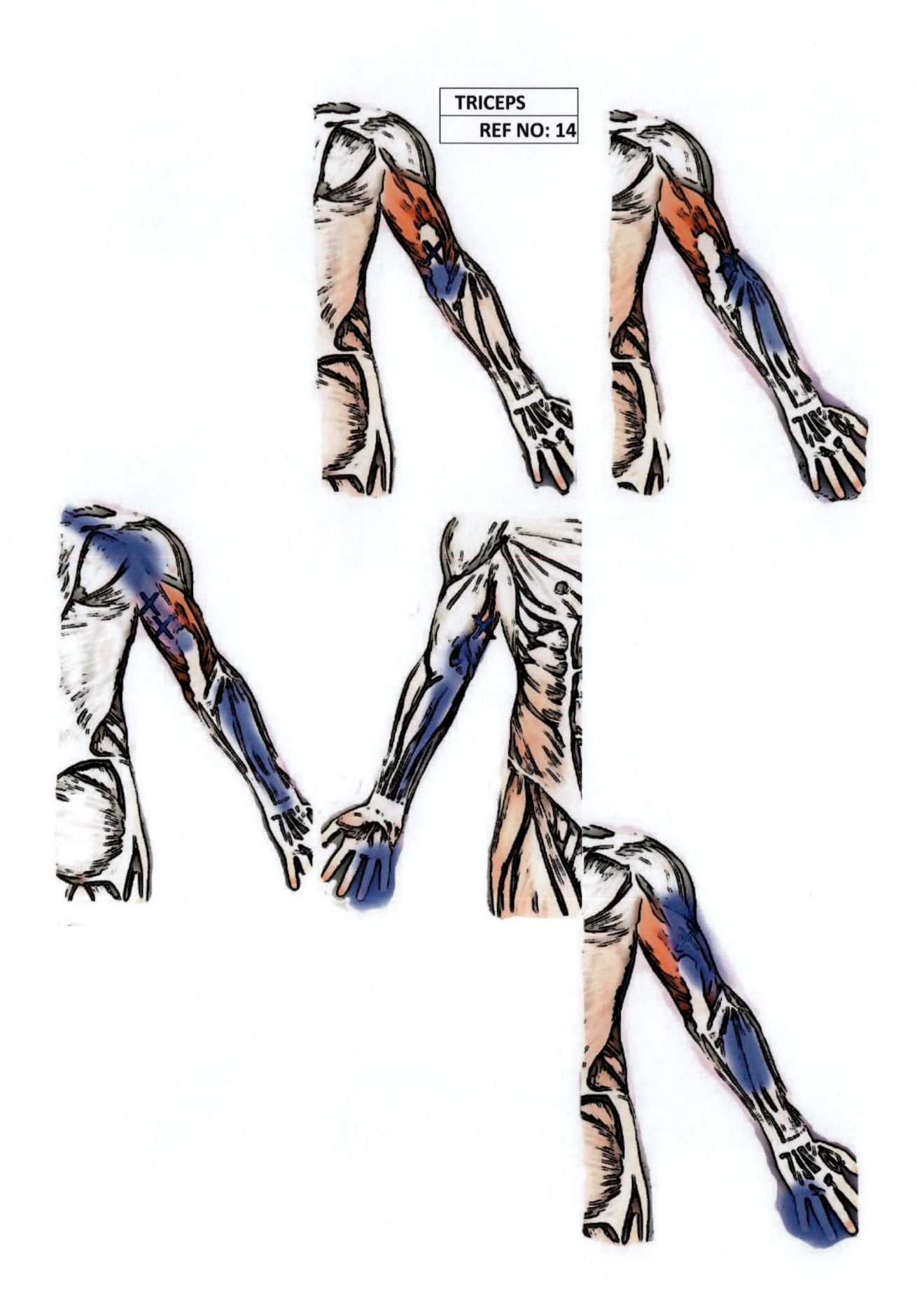

72

ILIOCOSTALIS
REF NO: 16

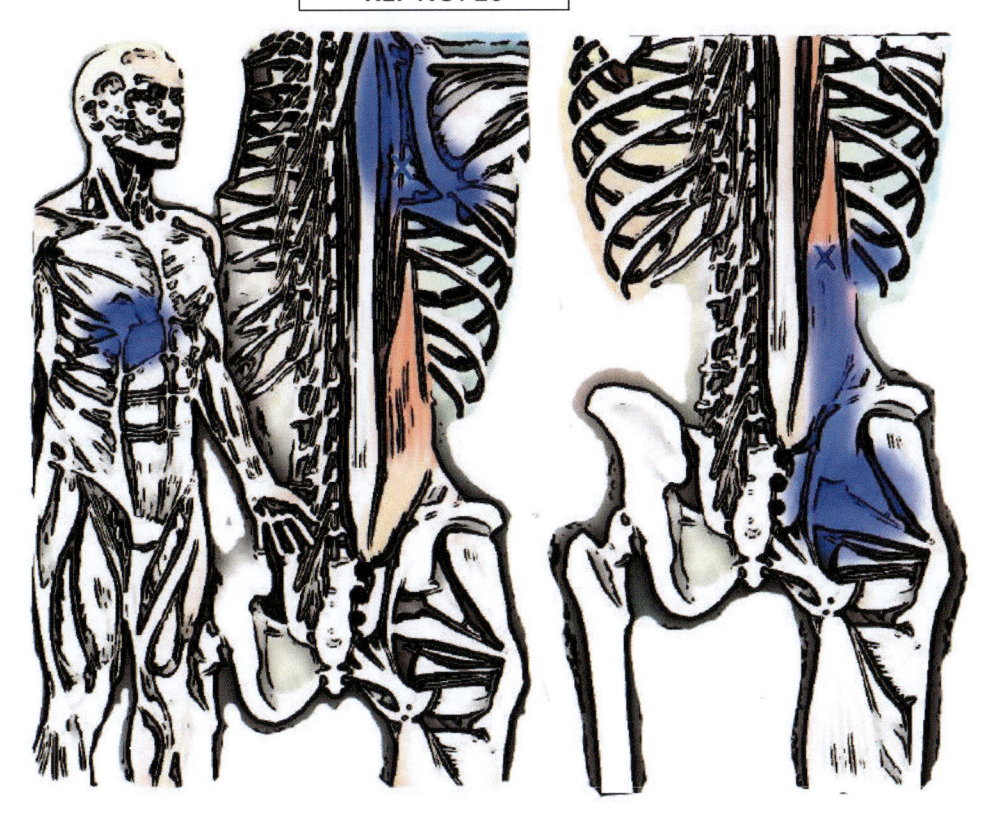

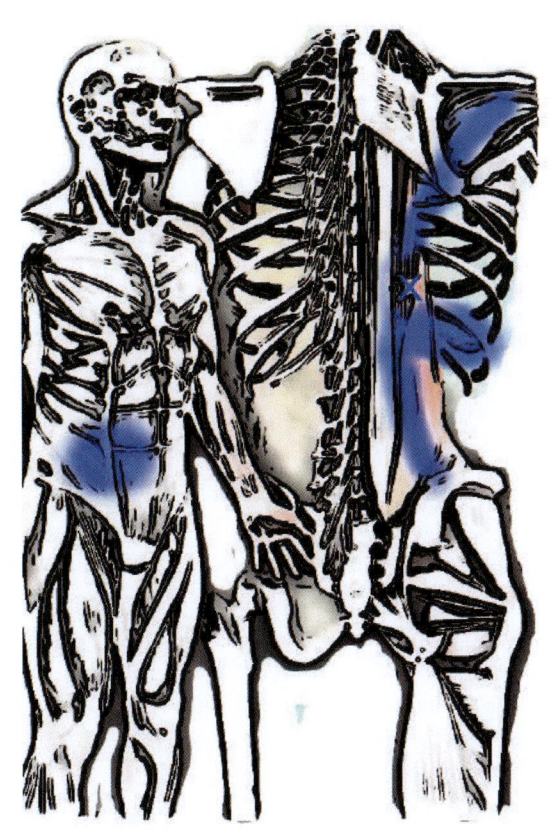

ARM PAIN REFERRAL CHART / DIAGRAMS

Location of Pain	Muscle	Referral	Picture Ref no:
Posterior Arm Pain, Posterior Forearm Pain, Anterior Arm Pain	Scalene Muscles	Trigger points in these muscles can refer in two finger-like projections into the chest. Other common patterns are into the shoulder, scapula and down the lateral arm, into the thumb and index finger. The Scalenes can impinge on the Brachial Plexus, causing nerve pain or numbness down the arm. This is called Thoracic Outlet Syndrome.	Ref no: 1
Posterior Arm Pain, Posterior Forearm Pain, Anterior Arm Pain	Triceps	The long head usually refers pain into the posterior shoulder and sometimes down into the posterior forearm (skipping the elbow). Trigger points in the center of the medial head refer into the Olecranon Process. The trigger points in the lateral part of the medial head refer to the lateral epicondyle, and are a common component of "Tennis Elbow".	Ref no: 2
Posterior Arm Pain, Anterior Arm Pain	Deltoid	Trigger points in the anterior Deltoid refer into the anterior and lateral shoulder. Trigger points in the posterior Deltoid refer into the posterior shoulder with spillover down the lateral arm.	Ref no: 3
Posterior Arm Pain	Subscapularis	The Subscapularis primarily refers to the posterior shoulder with spillover into the posterior medial arm and both sides of the wrist.	Ref no: 4
Posterior Arm Pain, Anterior Arm Pain	Supraspinatus	The primary referral is a deep ache in the mid deltoid area, with spillover down the arm into the elbow.	Ref no: 5
Posterior Arm Pain, Posterior Forearm Pain	Teres Major	Primary referral is deep in the posterior deltoid region, with spillover infrequently into the dorsal part of the forearm.	Ref no: 6
Posterior Arm Pain	Teres Minor	Pain is referred into the posterior deltoid, and down the posterior arm.	Ref no: 7
Posterior Arm Pain	Latissimus Dorsi	The main trigger point location for this muscle refers pain into the inferior scapular area, with spillover down the posterior arm and hand. An unusual trigger point in the anterior mid muscle refers pain inferiorly and sometimes into the anterior shoulder.	Ref no: 8

Posterior Arm Pain, Posterior Forearm Pain	Coracobrachialis	Trigger points in this muscle refer pain into the lateral shoulder, and down into the dorsal arm, skipping the elbow and wrist.	Ref no: 9
Posterior Forearm Pain	Extensor Carpi Radialis Longus	Trigger points in this muscle refer primarily to the lateral epicondyle. Secondary referral can be in the anatomical snuff box – between the thumb and first finger. Spillover referral is down the posterior arm.	Ref no: 10
Posterior Forearm Pain	Extensor Carpi Radialis Brevis	Trigger points in this muscle refer to the posterior wrist. This is one of the most common myofascial causes of pain in the back of the wrist.	Ref no: 11
Anterior Forearm Pain	Palmaris Longus	The referral pain of this muscle is a superficial needle-like prickling pain, rather than the deep aching of most other muscles. The primary location is into the palm, with spillover up into the forearm.	Ref no: 12
Anterior Forearm Pain	Pronator Teres	Trigger points in this muscle refer deep into the wrist and anterior forearm.	Ref no: 13
Anterior Forearm Pain	Serratus Anterior	The primary referral pattern is locally around the trigger point, but spillover may also occur down the Ulnar side of the arm. Also this spot can refer to the scapula.	Ref no: 14
Anterior Arm Pain	Infraspinatus	The main referral pattern is deep into the anterior shoulder joint, with spillover down the anterior side of the arm. Less common trigger points near the lower medial border refer pain into the Rhomboids.	Ref no: 15
Anterior Arm Pain	Biceps Brachii	The main referral pattern is up into the shoulder, with spillover into the posterior aspect above the scapula. A less common referral is into the anterior elbow and forearm.	Ref no: 16
Anterior Arm Pain	Brachialis	The main referral is into the thumb, with secondary patterns in the anterior arm and anterior elbow joint.	Ref no: 17

ARM PAIN CHART DIAGRAMS

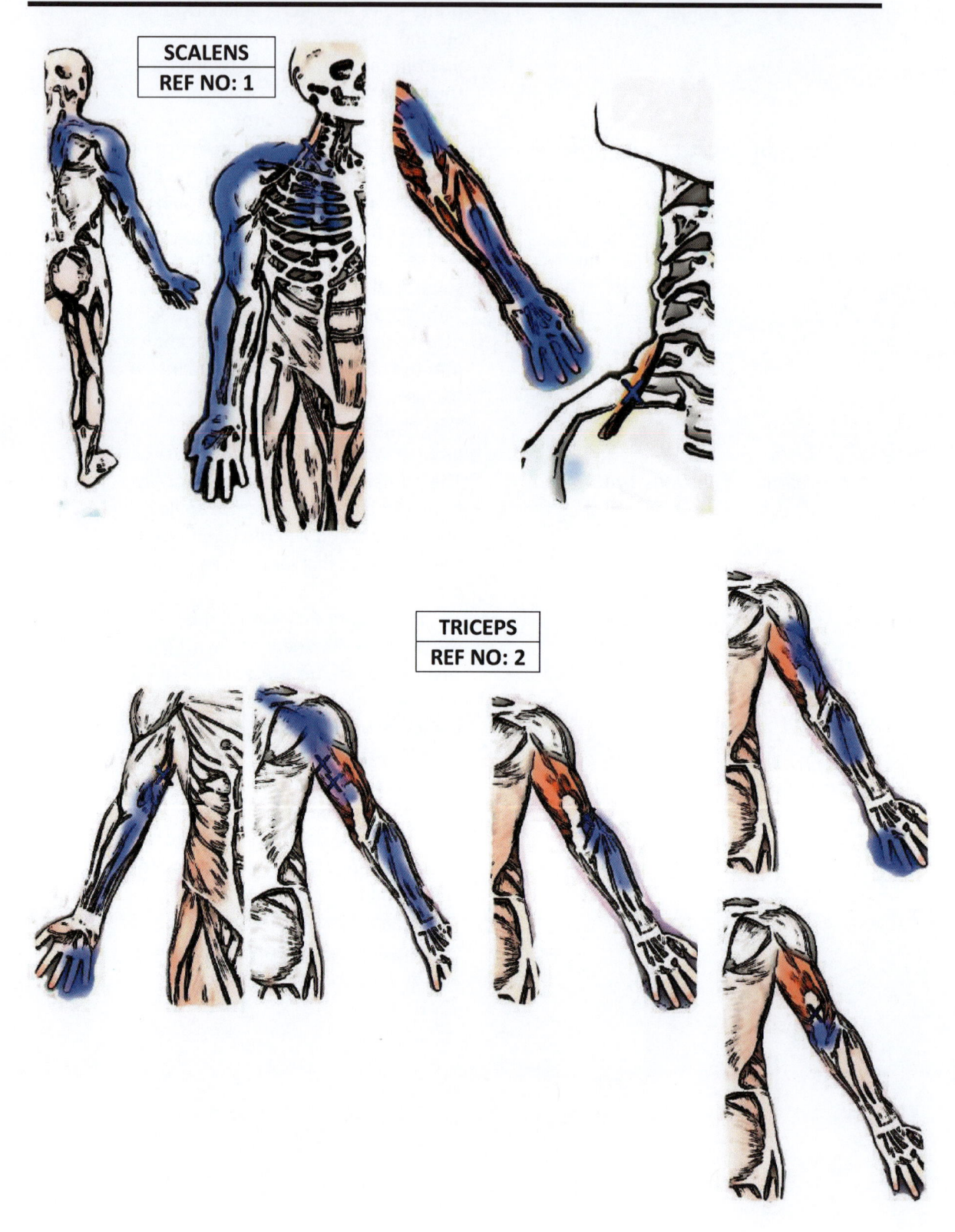

SCALENS
REF NO: 1

TRICEPS
REF NO: 2

DELTOIDS
REF NO: 3

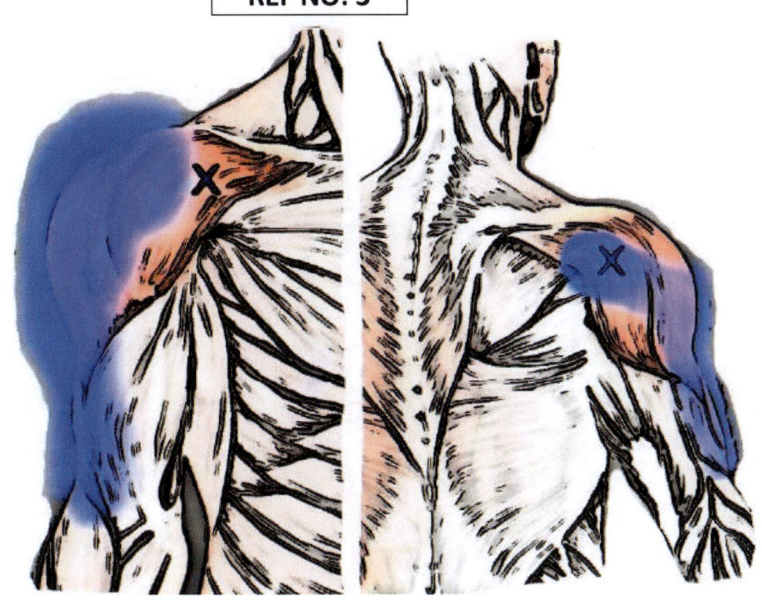

SUBSCAPULARIS
REF NO: 4

SUPRASPINATUS
REF NO: 5

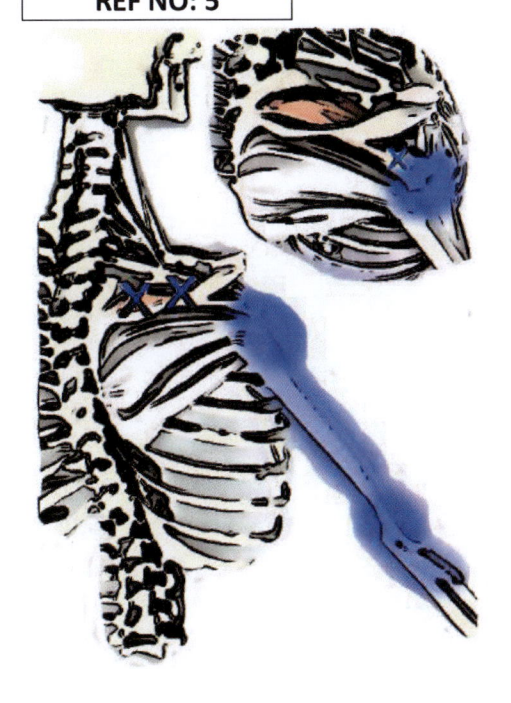

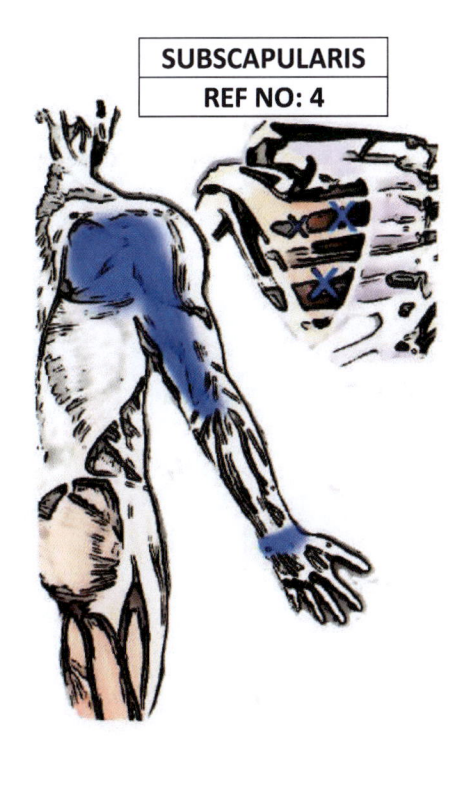

TERES MINOR
REF NO: 7

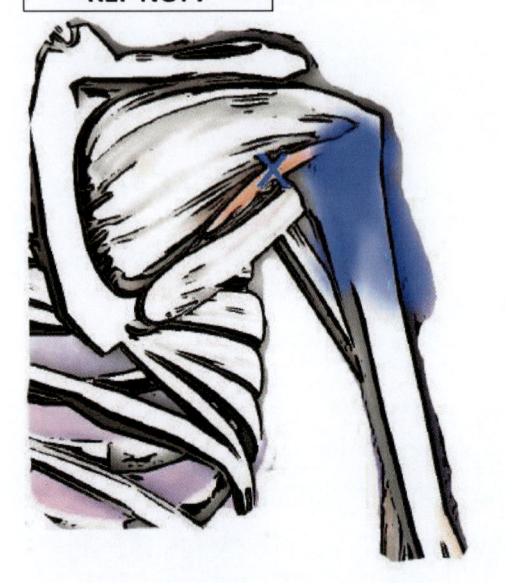

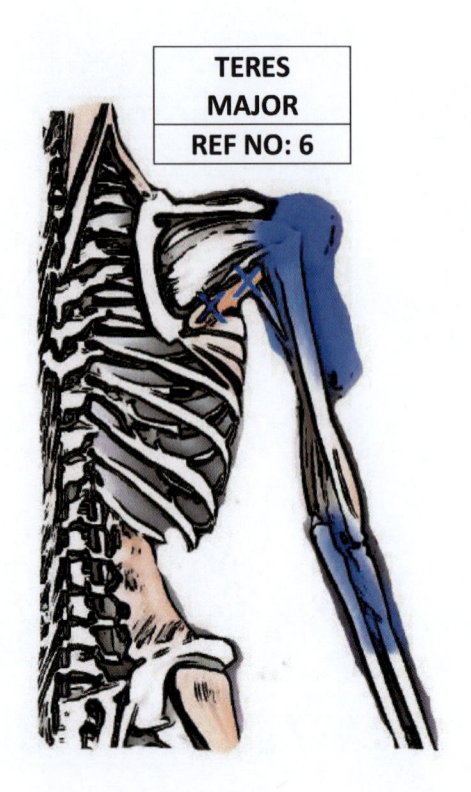

TERES MAJOR
REF NO: 6

LATISSIMUS DORSI
REF NO: 8

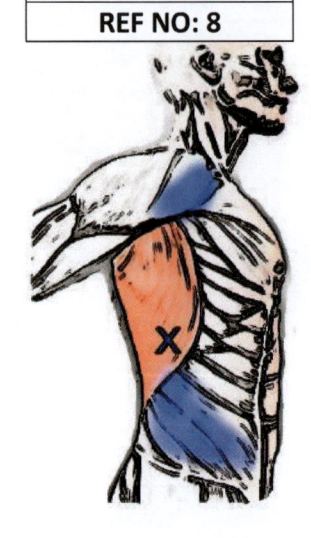

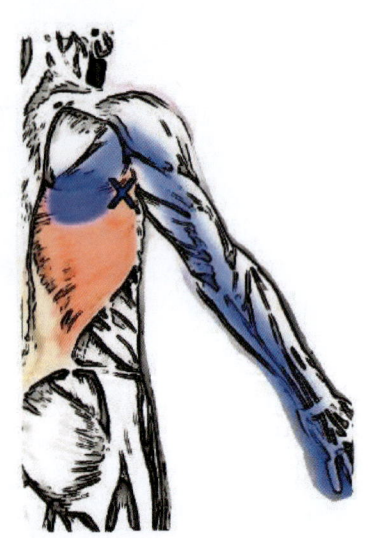

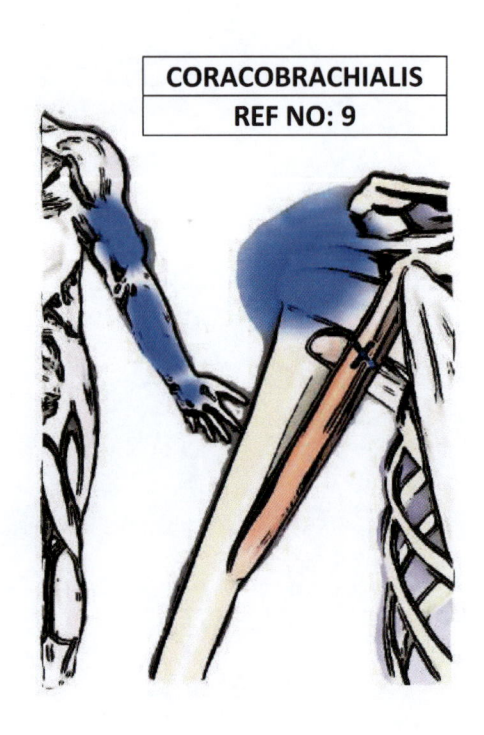

CORACOBRACHIALIS
REF NO: 9

EXTENSOR CARPI RADIALIS LONGUS
REF NO: 10

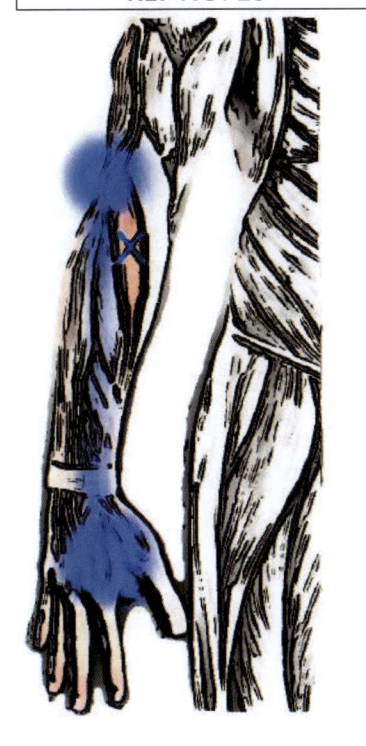

EXTENSOR CARPI RADIALIS BREVIS
REF NO: 11

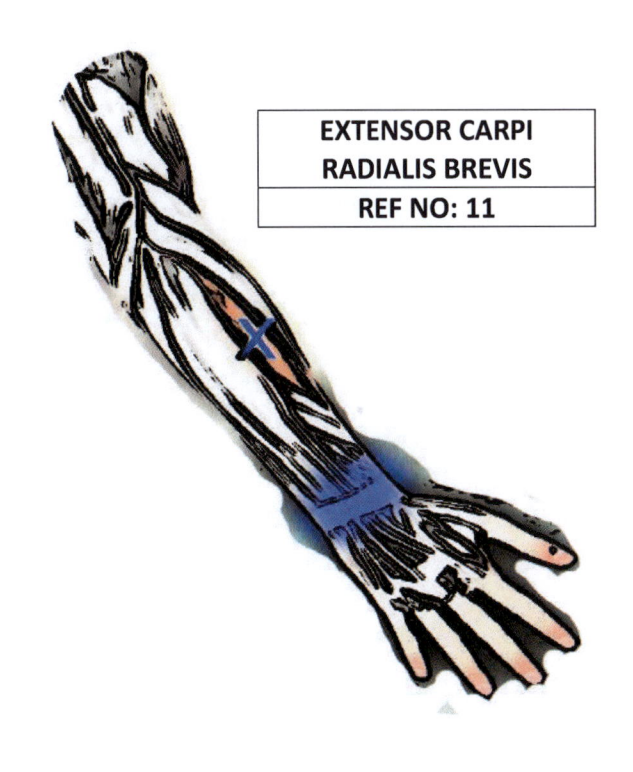

PRONATOR TERES
REF NO: 13

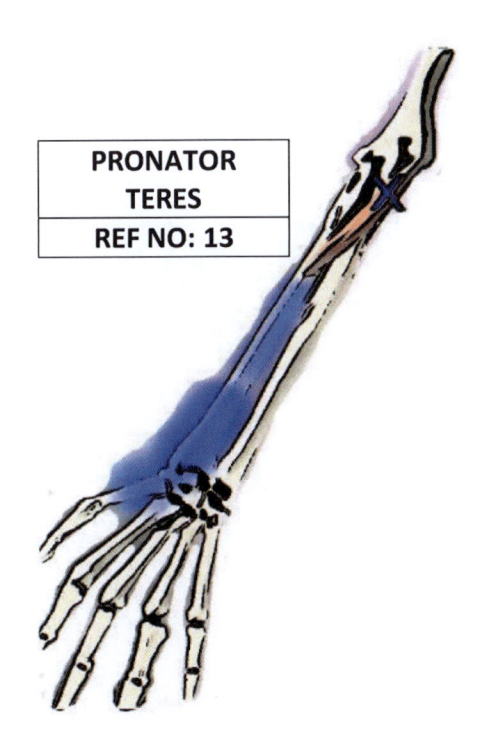

PALMARIS LONGUS
REF NO: 12

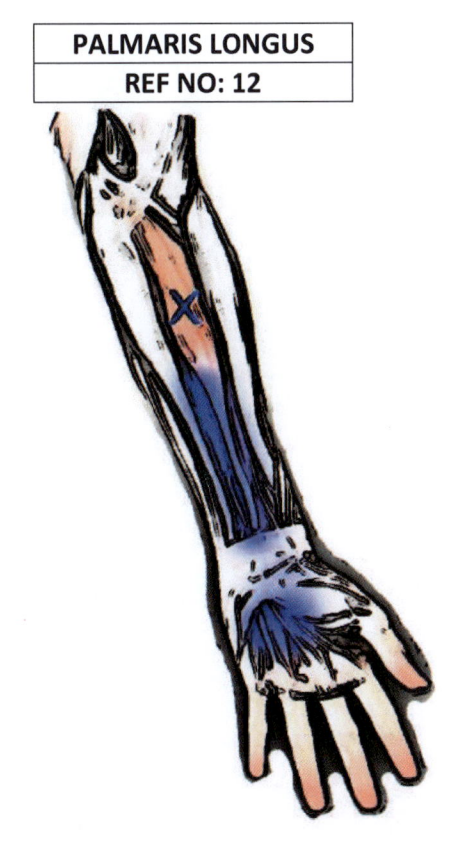

SERRATUS ANTERIOR
REF NO: 14

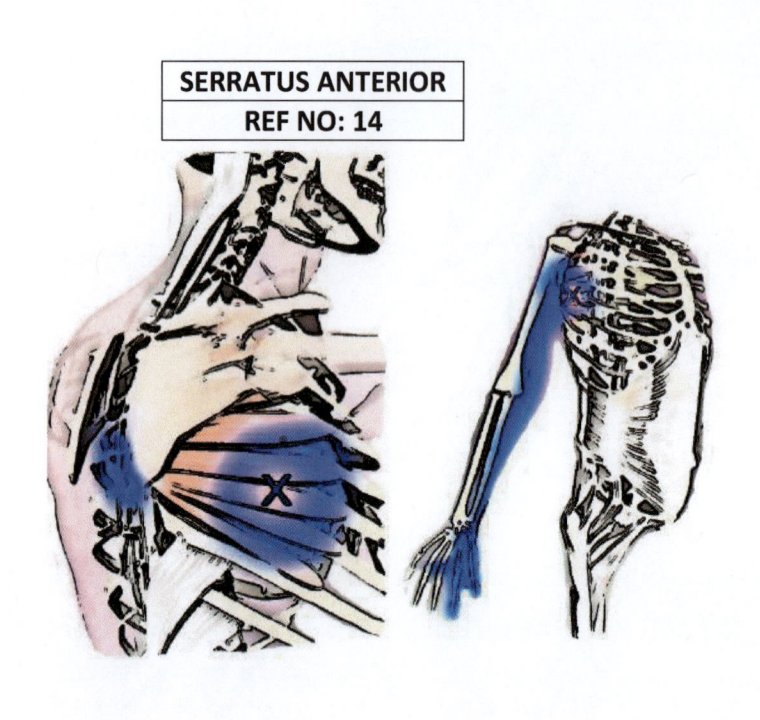

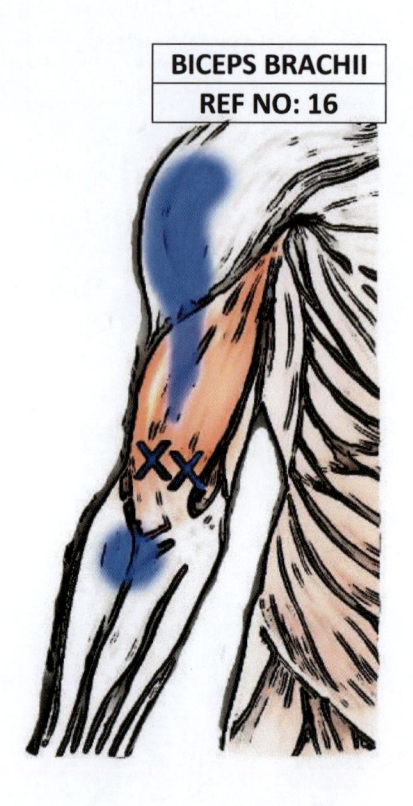

BICEPS BRACHII
REF NO: 16

INFRASPINATUS
REF NO: 15

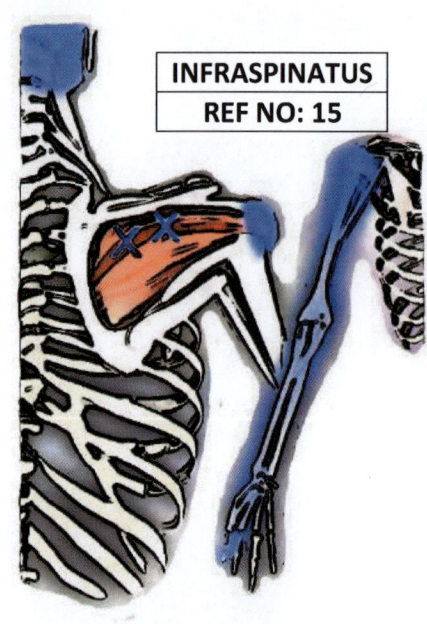

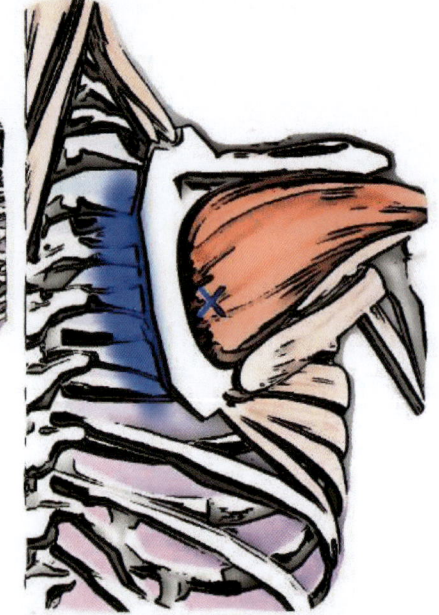

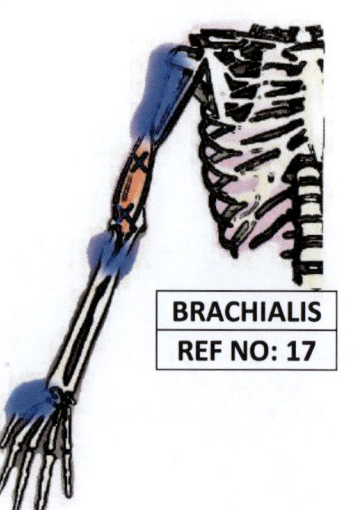

BRACHIALIS
REF NO: 17

WRIST PAIN REFERRAL CHART / DIAGRAMS

Location of Pain	Muscle	Referral	Picture Ref no:
Posterior Wrist Pain	Extensor Carpi Radialis Brevis	Trigger points in this muscle refer to the posterior wrist. This is one of the most common myofascial causes of pain in the back of the wrist.	Ref no: 1
Posterior Wrist Pain	Extensor Carpi Radialis Longus	Trigger points in this muscle refer primarily to the lateral epicondyle. Secondary referral can be in the anatomical snuff box – between the thumb and first finger. Spillover referral is down the posterior arm.	Ref no: 2
Posterior Wrist Pain	Extensor Digitorum	Trigger points refer pain into the middle or second finger, with spillover down the dorsal aspect of the arm. Trigger points in the middle finger extensor are the most common. Trigger points in the ring finger extensor also refer pain into the lateral epicondyle.	Ref no: 3
Posterior Wrist Pain	Extensor Carpi Ulnaris	Trigger points refers into the posterior Ulnar side of the wrist	Ref no: 4
Posterior Wrist Pain	Subscapularis	The Subscapularis primarily refers to the posterior shoulder with spillover into the posterior medial arm and both sides of the wrist.	Ref no: 5
Posterior Wrist Pain	Coracobrachialis	Trigger points in this muscle refer pain into the lateral shoulder, and down into the dorsal arm, skipping the elbow and wrist.	Ref no: 6
Posterior Wrist Pain, Anterior Wrist Pain	Latissimus Dorsi	The main trigger point location for this muscle refers pain into the inferior scapular area, with spillover down the posterior arm and hand. An unusual trigger point in the anterior mid muscle refers pain inferiorly and sometimes into the anterior shoulder.	Ref no: 7

Anterior Wrist Pain	Flexor Carpi Ulnaris	Trigger points refer to pain into the Ulnar side of the wrist	Ref no: 8
Anterior Wrist Pain	Opponens Pollicis	Trigger points in this muscle refer pain into the thumb and base of the wrist	Ref no: 9
Anterior Wrist Pain	Pectoralis Major	Trigger points in the clavicular section refer into the anterior shoulder. Points in the sternal section refer intense pain into the anterior chest and medial aspect of the arm. Points in the costal and abdominal sections of the muscle refer into the breast, causing breast tenderness and nipple hypersensitivity.	Ref no: 10
Anterior Wrist Pain	Pectoralis Minor	Primary referral pattern is over the anterior chest and shoulder, with spillover down the medial side of the arm.	Ref no: 11
Anterior Wrist Pain	Palmaris Longus	The referral pain of this muscle is a superficial needle-like prickling pain, rather than the deep aching of most other muscles. The primary location is into the palm, with spillover up the forearm.	Ref no: 12
Anterior Wrist Pain	Pronator Teres	Trigger points in this muscle refer deep into the wrist and anterior forearm.	Ref no: 13
Anterior Wrist Pain	Serratus Anterior	The primary referral pattern is locally around the trigger point, but spillover can occur down the Ulnar side of the arm. Also this spot can refer to the scapula.	Ref no: 14

WRIST PAIN CHART DIAGRAMS

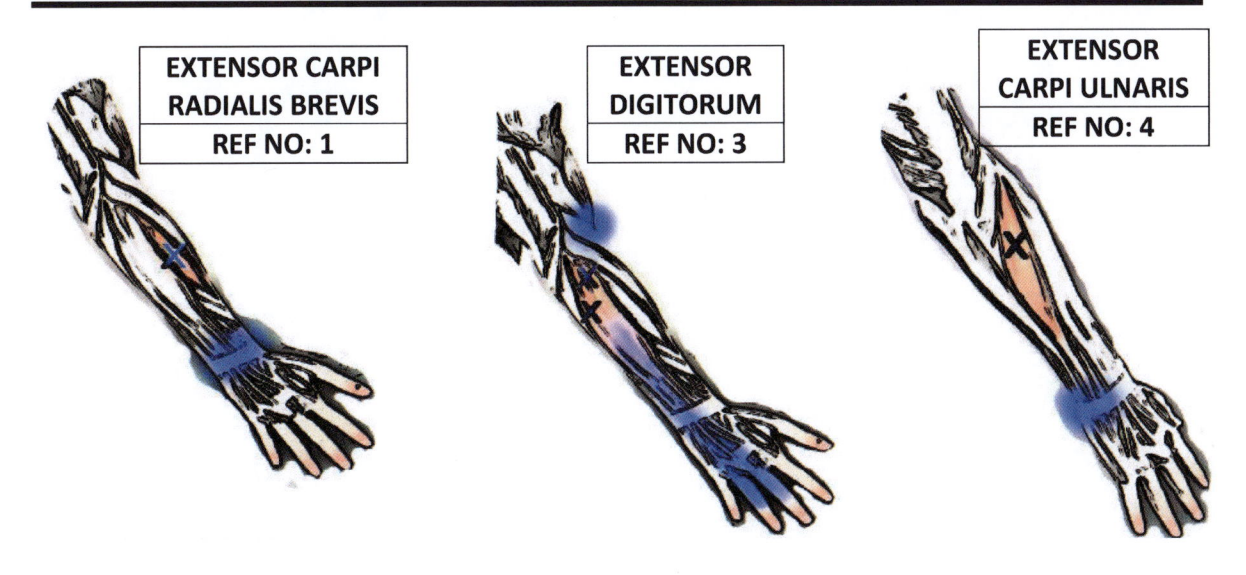

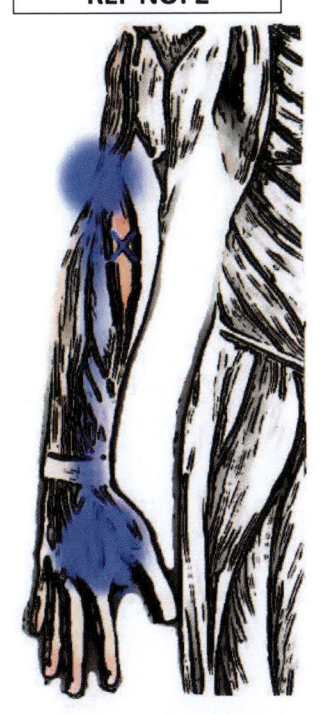

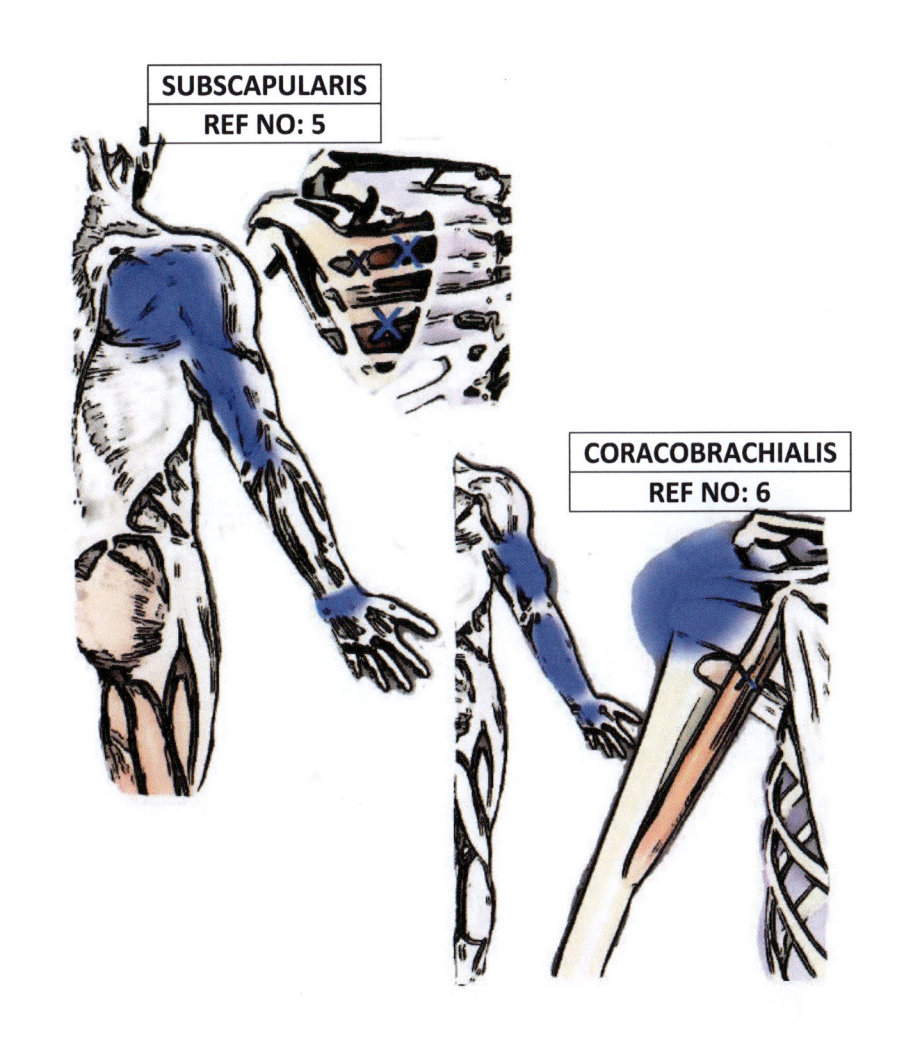

EXTENSOR CARPI RADIALIS BREVIS
REF NO: 1

EXTENSOR DIGITORUM
REF NO: 3

EXTENSOR CARPI ULNARIS
REF NO: 4

EXTENSOR CARPI RADIALIS LONGUS
REF NO: 2

SUBSCAPULARIS
REF NO: 5

CORACOBRACHIALIS
REF NO: 6

LATISSIMUS DORSI
REF NO: 7

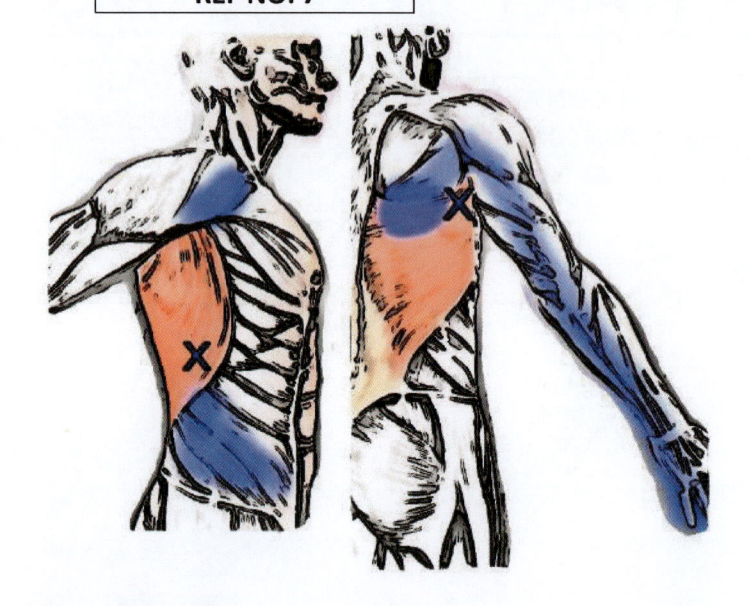

FLEXOR CARPI ULNARIS
REF NO: 8

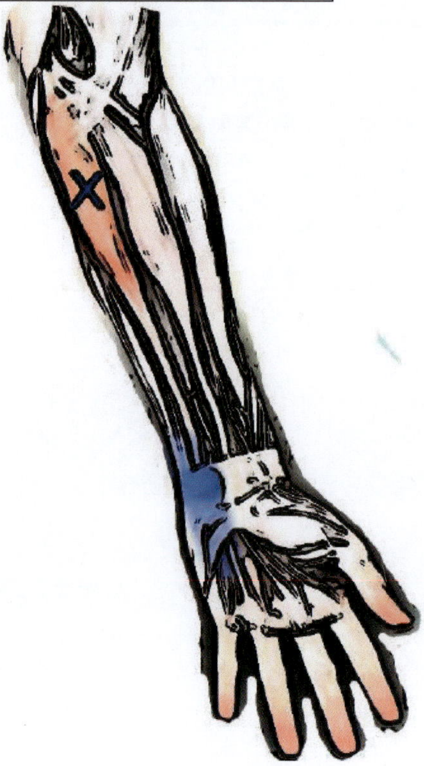

OPPONENS POLLICIS
REF NO: 9

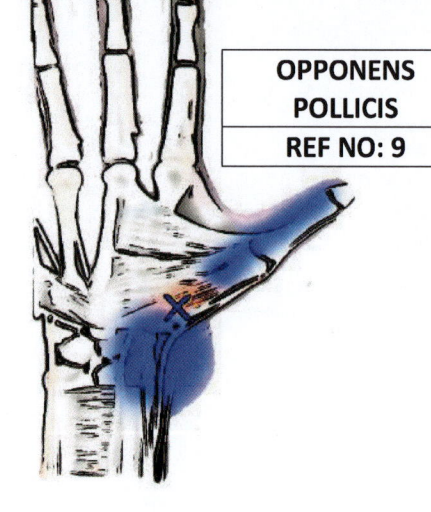

PECTORALIS MAJOR
REF NO: 10

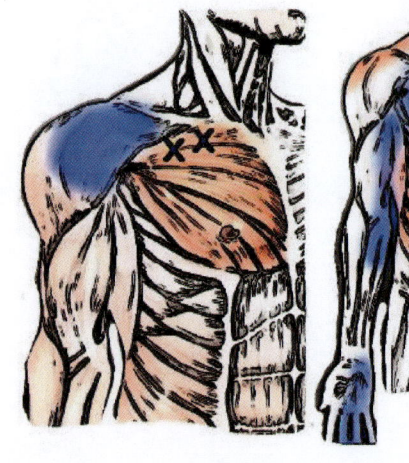

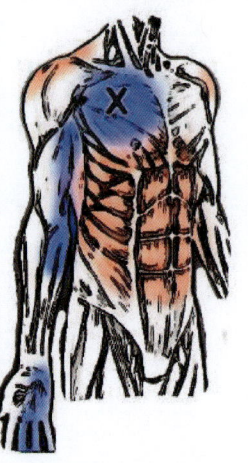

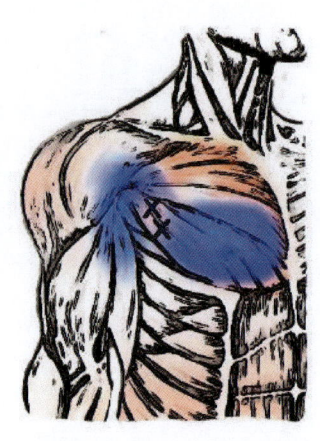

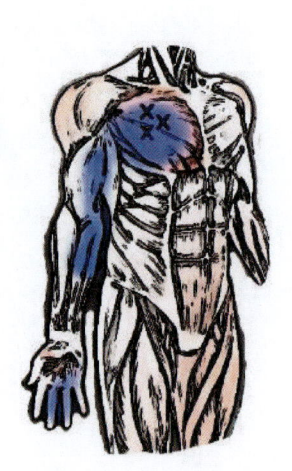

| PECTORALIS MINOR |
| REF NO: 11 |

| PALMARIS LONGUS |
| REF NO: 12 |

| PRONATOR TERES |
| REF NO: 13 |

| SERRATUS ANTERIOR |
| REF NO: 14 |

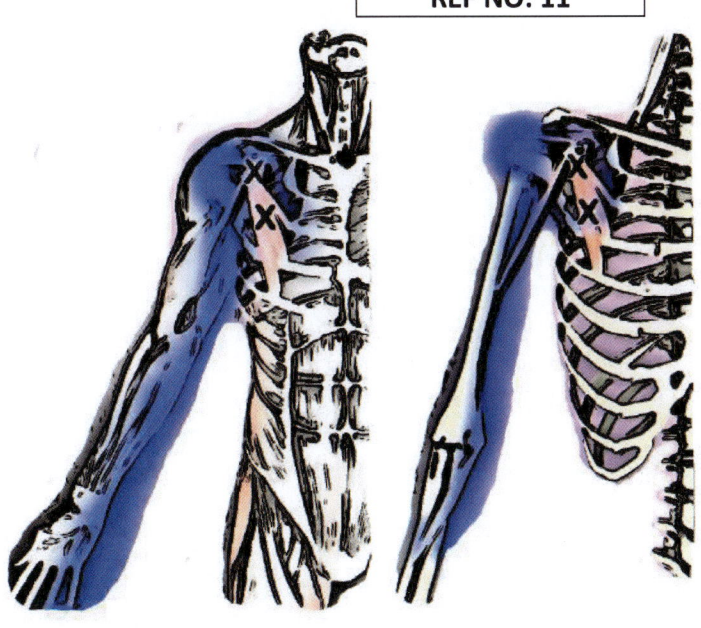

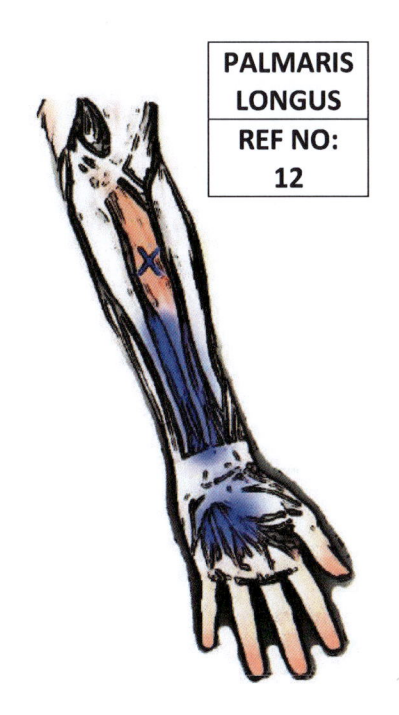

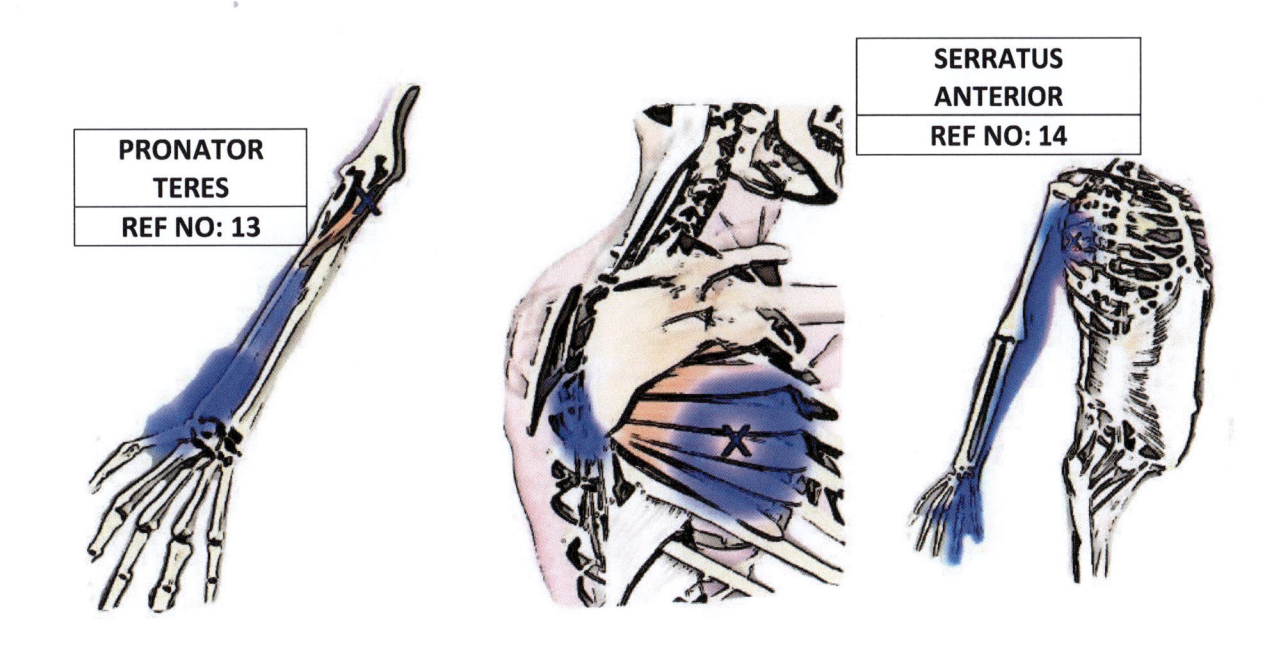

ANTERIOR SHOULDER PAIN REFERRAL CHART / DIAGRAMS

Location of Pain	Muscle	Referral	Picture Ref no:
Anterior Shoulder Pain	Infraspinatus	The main referral pattern is deep into the anterior shoulder joint, with spillover down the anterior side of the arm. Less common trigger points near the lower medial border refer pain into the Rhomboids.	Ref no: 1
Anterior Shoulder Pain	Deltoid	Trigger points in the anterior Deltoid refer into the anterior and lateral shoulder. Trigger points in the posterior Deltoid refer into the posterior shoulder with spillover down the lateral side of the arm.	Ref no: 2
Anterior Shoulder Pain	Scalene Muscles	Trigger points in these muscles can refer in two finger-like projections into the chest. Other common patterns are into the shoulder, scapula and down the lateral arm, into the thumb and index finger. The Scalenes can impinge on the Brachial Plexus, causing nerve pain or numbness down the arm. This is called Thoracic Outlet Syndrome.	Ref no: 3
Anterior Shoulder Pain	Supraspinatus	The primary referral is a deep ache in the mid deltoid area, with spillover down the arm and into the elbow.	Ref no: 4
Anterior Shoulder Pain	Pectoralis Major	Trigger points in the clavicular section refer into the anterior shoulder. Points in the sternal section refer intense pain into the anterior chest and medial aspect of the arm. Points in the costal and abdominal sections of the muscle refer into the breast, causing breast tenderness and nipple hypersensitivity.	Ref no: 5
Anterior Shoulder Pain	Pectoralis Minor	Primary referral pattern is over the anterior chest and shoulder, with spillover down the medial arm.	Ref no: 6
Anterior Shoulder Pain	Biceps Brachii	The main referral pattern is up into the shoulder, with spillover into the posterior aspect above the scapula. A less common referral is into the anterior elbow and forearm.	Ref no: 7
Anterior Shoulder Pain	Coracobrachialis	Trigger points in this muscle refer pain into the lateral shoulder, and down into the dorsal arm, skipping the elbow and wrist.	Ref no: 8

| Anterior Shoulder Pain | Latissimus Dorsi | The main trigger point location for this muscle refers pain into the inferior scapular area, with spillover down the posterior side of the arm and hand. An unusual trigger point in the anterior mid muscle refers pain inferiorly and sometimes into the anterior shoulder. | Ref no: 9 |

ANTERIOR SHOULDER PAIN CHART DIAGRAMS

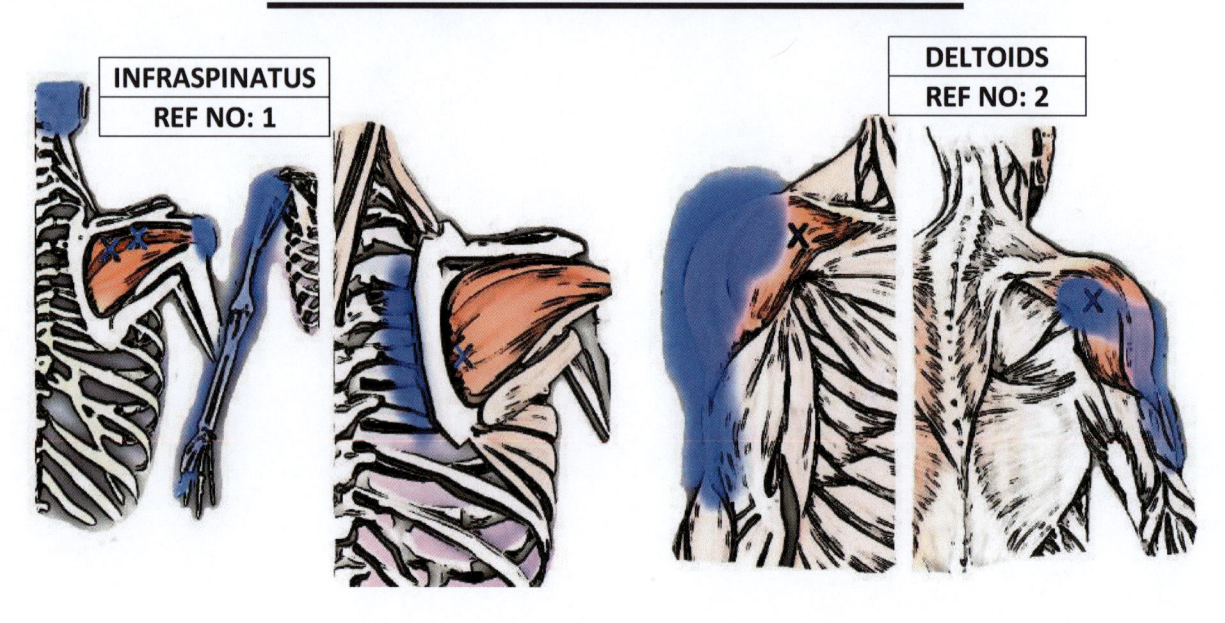

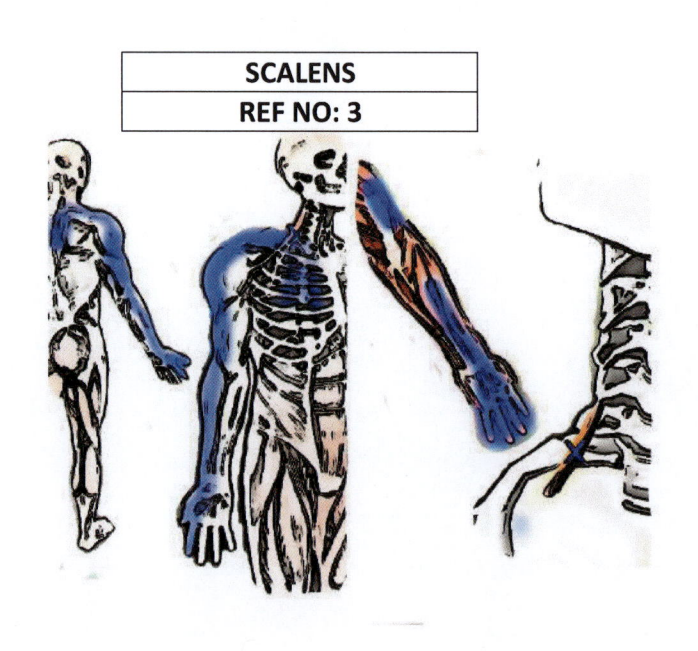

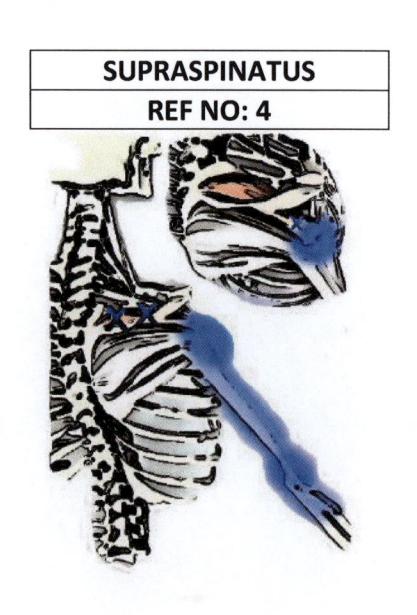

INFRASPINATUS
REF NO: 1

DELTOIDS
REF NO: 2

SCALENS
REF NO: 3

SUPRASPINATUS
REF NO: 4

88

PECTORALIS MAJOR
REF NO: 5

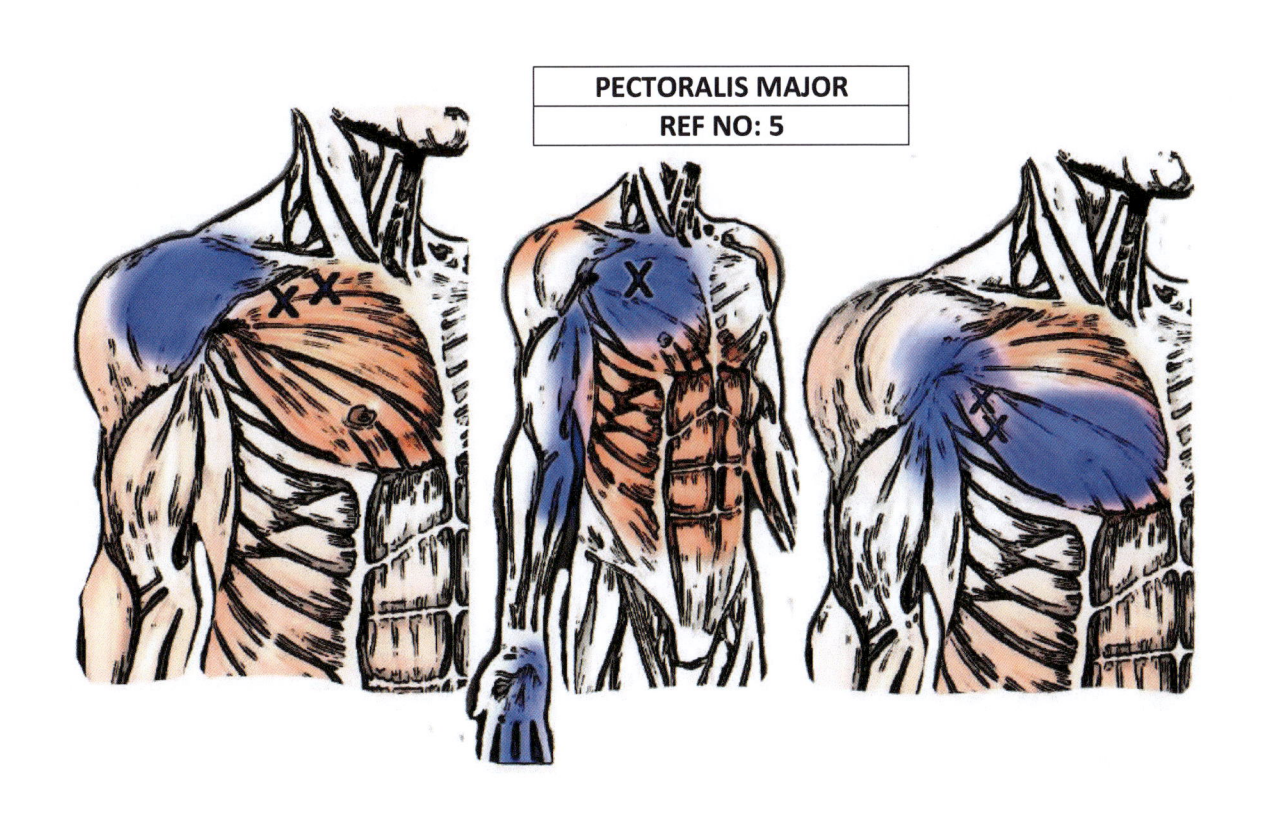

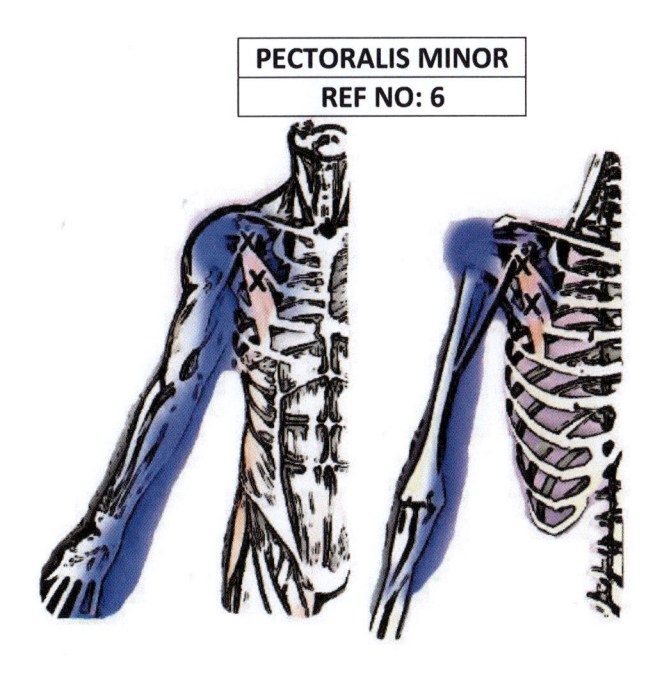

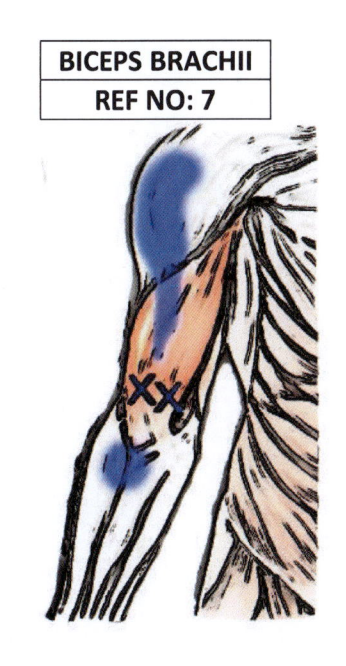

PECTORALIS MINOR
REF NO: 6

BICEPS BRACHII
REF NO: 7

CORACOBRACHIALIS
REF NO: 8

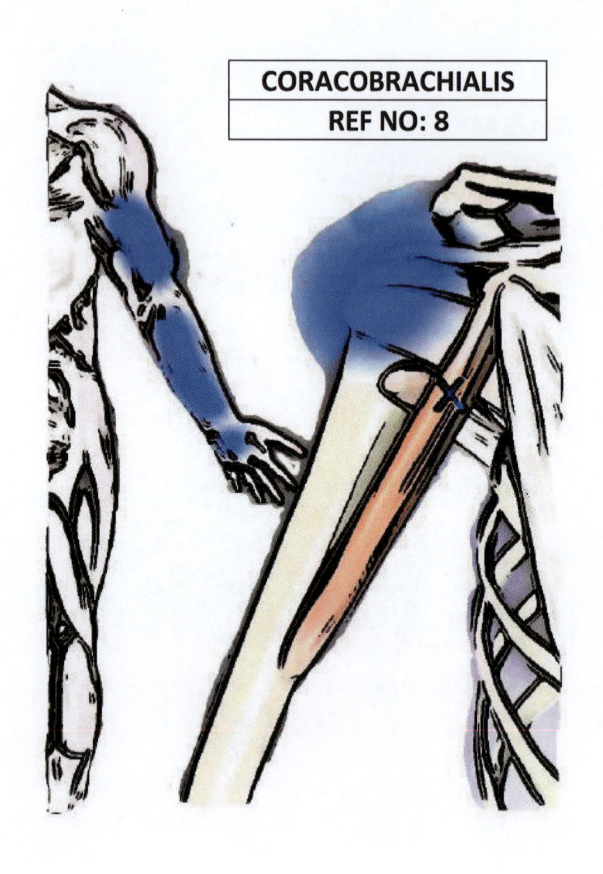

LATISSIMUS DORSI
REF NO: 9

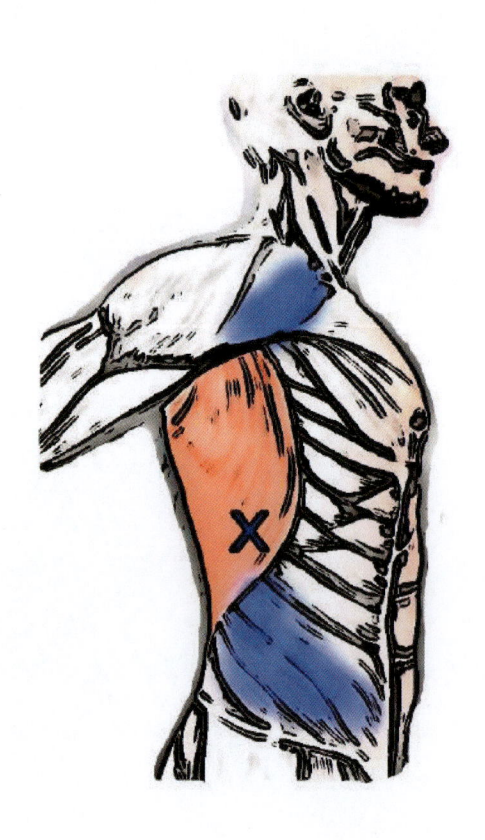

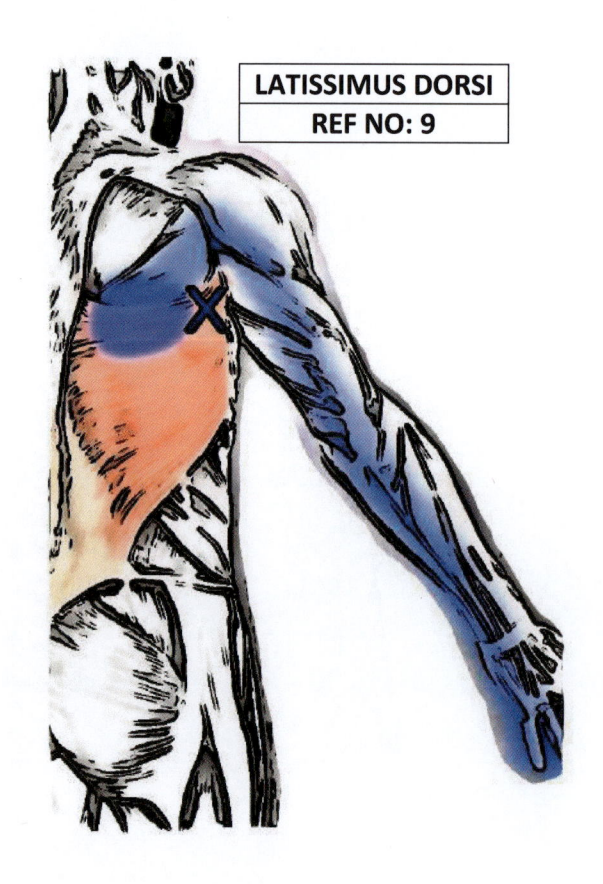

HEADACHE PAIN REFERRAL CHART / DIAGRAMS

Location of Pain	Muscle	Referral	Picture Ref no:
Temporal Headache, Posterior Headache	Trapezius	Trigger points on the lateral upper edge refer into lateral neck and temples, causing "tension neck ache". Other points in the middle and lower fibres refer into the posterior neck and shoulders.	Ref no: 1
Temporal Headache, Frontal Headache, Posterior Headache	Sternocleidomastoid	Trigger points in the sternal (superficial) division refer to the cheek and along the supraorbital ridge. The lowest points refer down into the sternum. The highest points refer to the occipital ridge and vertex of the head. Trigger points in the costal (deep) division refer to the forehead. The most superior trigger points refer into the ear, and can cause postural dizziness.	Ref no: 2
Temporal Headache, Posterior Headache	Temporalis	Trigger points refer into the teeth causing hypersensitivity, and into and above the eye and temple, causing headaches.	Ref no: 3
Temporal Headache, Posterior Headache	Splenius Cervicis	The lower trigger point refers pain into the angle of the neck. The upper trigger point shoots pain from the inside of the head to the back of the eye.	Ref no: 4
Temporal Headache, Posterior Headache	Suboccipitals	Trigger points in these muscles cause head pain that penetrates the skull but is difficult to localise. Patients are likely to describe it as "all over", including the occiput, eye and forehead, but without any clarity. Includes 4 muscles – Rectus Capitis Posterior Minor, Rectus Capitis Posterior Major, Obliquus Capitis Superior and Obliquus Capitis Inferior.	Ref no: 5
Temporal Headache, Frontal Headache, Posterior Headache	Semispinalis Capitis	Refers into the temple area with spillover into the lateral head	Ref no: 6

Frontal Headache	Frontalis	Forehead Headache	Ref no: 7
Frontal Headache	Zygomaticus Major	The trigger points in this muscle refer pain in an arc up the side of the nose and end near the forehead.	Ref no: 8
Posterior Headache	Occipitalis	Headache in the posterior lateral part of the head, plus pain behind the eye	Ref no: 9

HEADACHE PAIN CHART DIAGRAMS

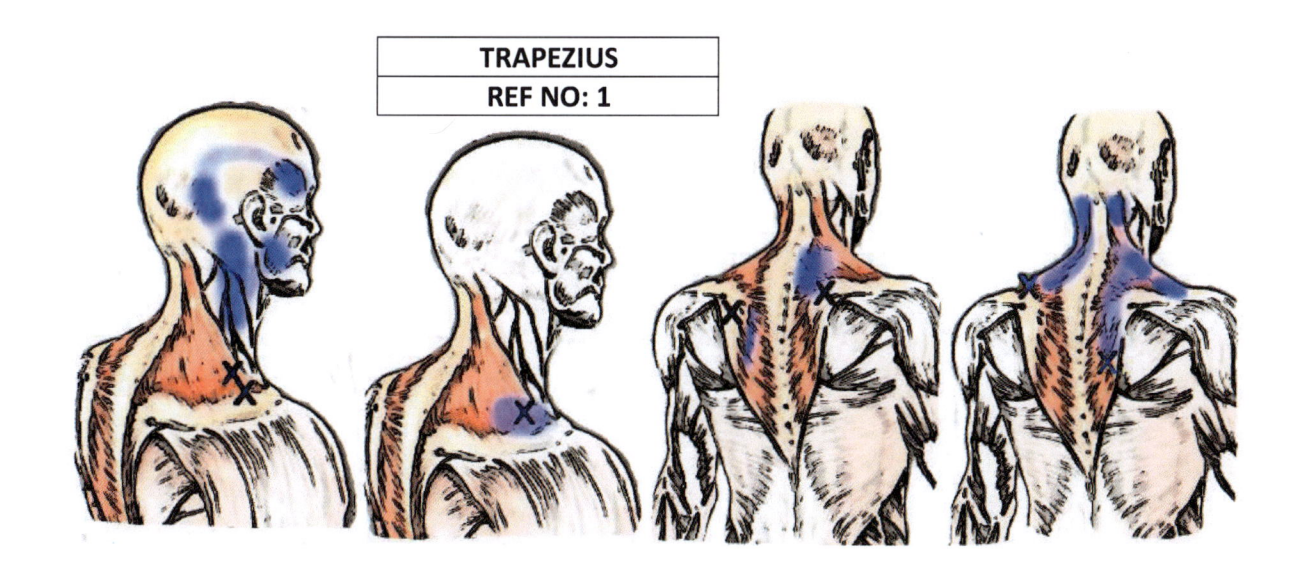

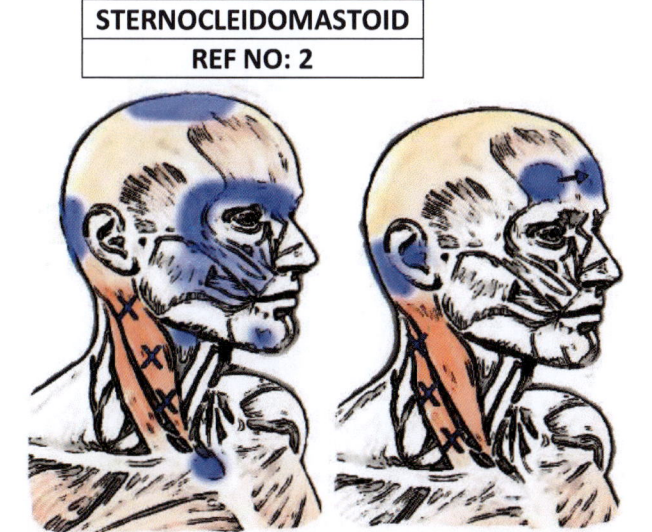

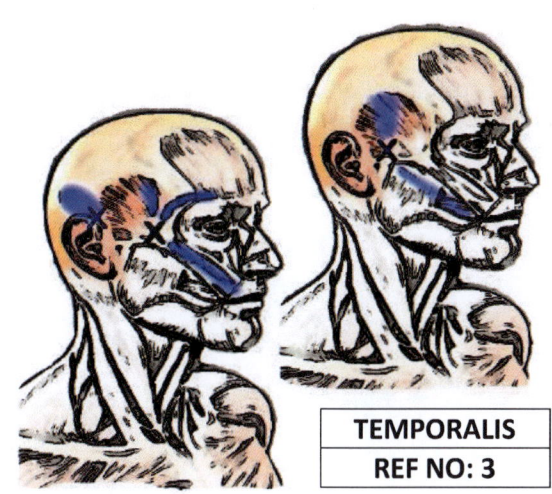

TRAPEZIUS
REF NO: 1

STERNOCLEIDOMASTOID
REF NO: 2

TEMPORALIS
REF NO: 3

SPLENIUS CERVICIES
REF NO: 4

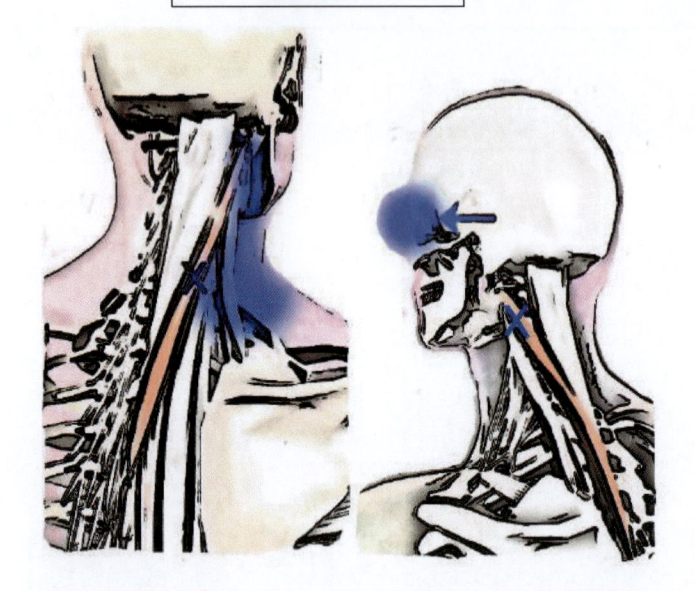

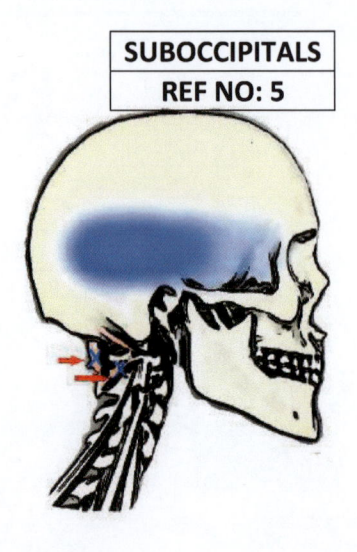

SUBOCCIPITALS
REF NO: 5

SEMISPINALIS CAPTIS
REF NO: 6

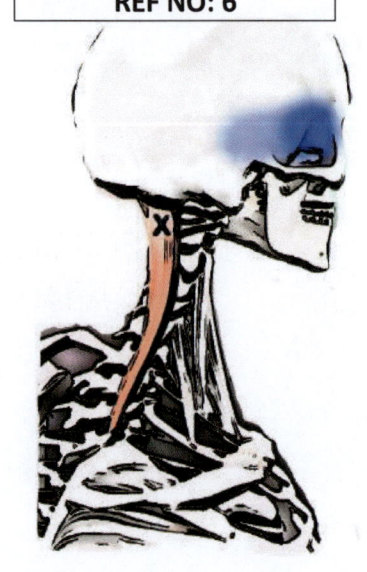

FRONTALIS
REF NO: 7

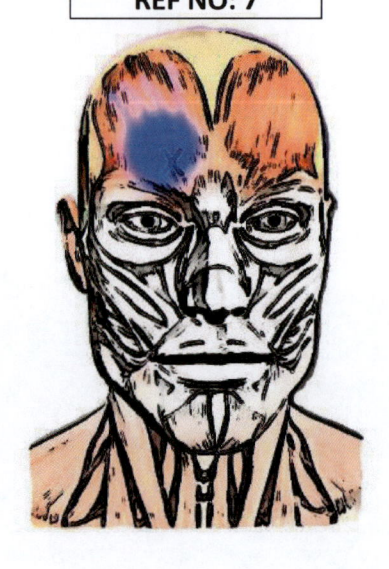

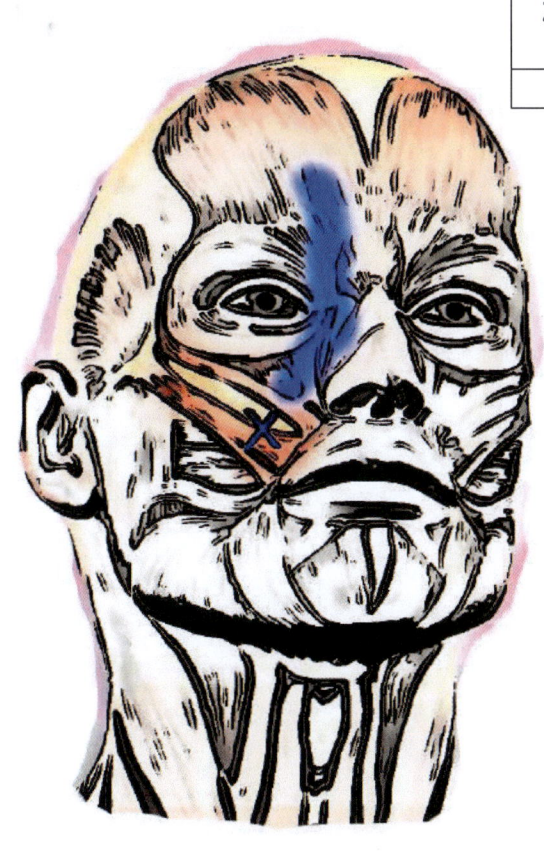

ZYGOMATICUS MAJOR
REF NO: 8

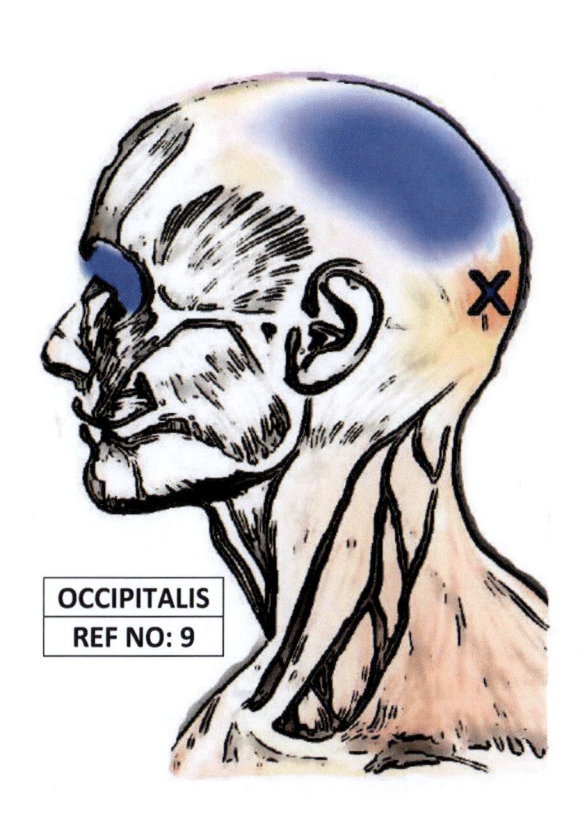

OCCIPITALIS
REF NO: 9

R.O.M.T: Range Of Motion Testing

R.O.M.T (CX) CERVICAL SPINE

MOVEMENT	RANGE	KEY MUSCLES AFFECTED BY R.O.M
FLEXION	45-50°	Neck extensors and trapezius
EXTENSION	85°	Neck flexors and sternocleidomastoid
LATERAL FLEXION	20-45°	Trapezius, SCM, splenius capitis, longissimus capitis, semispinalis
ROTATION	70-90°	Trapezius, SCM, splenius capitis, obliquus capitis inferior, semispinalis capitis, longissimus capitis

ORTHOPAEDIC TESTING OF THE CERVICAL SPINE (CX)

Test 1: MAXIMAL CERVICAL COMPRESSION TEST

Why do we do the test?	You will do the Maximal Cervical Compression Test to examine and also to differentiate between 1. The Radicular pain, which may be due to the IVF (**Intervertebral Foramina**) encroachment or the nerve pressure 2. Localised pain, which may be due to infection, fracture, inflammation in the Cx or musculoskeletal dysfunction 3. To assess for facet dysfunction
How do we do the test?	1. Have the client seated in front of you 2. Perform the cervical compression in all movements of the Cx (cervical spine): Flexion, Extension, Lateral Flexion L & R and Rotation L & R 3. The combined movement of rotation and the lateral flexion is the most dramatic way of limiting IVF size (on the side of the rotation and the lateral flexion
What you don't want to find?	Radicular pain

Test 2: CERVICAL DISTRACTION TEST

Why do we do the test?	You will do the Cervical Distraction Test to confirm nerve root involvement. If the Cervical Distraction Test is negative, then you should suspect a musculoskeletal dysfunction
How do we do the test?	1. Have the client seated or in a supine position 2. With your hands cupping the chin anteriorly and the occiput posteriorly, then gradually apply axial traction to the cervical spine
What you don't want to find?	That the presenting radial pain is relieved

Test 3: SHOULDER ABDUCTION TEST (BAKODY'S TEST)

Why do we do the test?	You will do the Shoulder Abduction Test (Bakody's Test) to test for radicular symptoms, especially those involving the C4 or C5 nerve roots
How do we do the test?	1. Have the client in a sitting or have the client lying supine and then the therapist passively abducts the arm until the forearm rests on top of the clients head.
What you don't want to find?	A decrease or relief of the symptoms, which can indicate a cervical extradural compression problem. Such as a herniated disc or a nerve root compression

FUNCTIONAL SCREENING SEQUENCE
CERVICAL SPINE (CX)

	Test 1: SCAPULOHUMERAL RYTHM TEST
Why do we do the test?	To check for any dysfunctions that will be occurring at the gelnohumeral and the scapulothoracic joint and or the muscles related to these joints.
How do we do the test?	1. Have the client seated on the table in front of you 2. Have the client with their arms hanging down and their elbows flexed at 90°, have their thumbs pointing upwards and slowly abduct the shoulder horizontal 3. Check the muscle firing sequence by using visual observation and light palpation they perform the movement 4. Normal activation sequence will involve shoulder elevation and or superior movement of the scapula only after approximately 60° of abduction
What you don't want to find?	The will have direct implications for the neck and the shoulder dysfunction. If an abnormal appears it will be as flowed. 1. Shoulder elevation and or rotation or a superior movement or winging of the scapula will occur within the first 60° of shoulder abduction, which will indicate a shortness of the levator scapula and or the upper traps and a weakness of the lower and middle traps and serratus anterior
	Test 2: NECK FLEXION TEST
Why do we do the test?	To check for muscle dysfunctions in the cervical spine which may be causing headaches, neck and shoulder pain and/or possible TMJ dysfunction.
How do we do the test?	1. Have the client on the treatment table in a supine position, with a pillow under their head. 2. Standing beside the client at the level of their neck, have the client lift their head no more than 2cm and bring their chin to their chest. 3. Check the muscle firing sequence using visual observation and light palpation as they perform this movement. 4. Normal activation sequence occurs if the client is able to hold their chin tucked in whilst flexing the head/neck
What you don't want to find?	If the pattern is abnormal it would be as follows: 1. The chin pokes forward during the motion indicating short and/or overactive sternocleidomastoid and weakness of the deep neck flexors.
	Test 3: PUSH UP TEST
Why do we do the test?	To check for any dysfunctions that will be occurring at the scapula
How do we do the test?	1. Have the client prone in a push up position and then have them perform a push-up or lower themselves from a push-up position 2. Check the scapula from behind using visual observation and light palpation as they perform this movement 3. Normal activation sequence occurs if the scapula retracts during the movement without winging or shifting superiorly as the trunk is lowered
What you don't want to find?	If an abnormal pattern appears, it would be as follows: 1. Winging, superior shifting or rotation of the scapulae indicating weakness of the lower stabilisers of the scapulae (serratus anterior, middle and lower trapezius).

R.O.M.T (TX) THORACIC SPINE MOTION TEST

MOVEMENT	RANGE	KEY MUSCLES AFFECTED BY R.O.M
FLEXION	30-40°	Tx Erector spinae, multifidis, rotatores
EXTENSION	0-25°	Rectus abdominis, internal and external obliques, transverse abdominis
LATERAL FLEXION	20-35°	Contralateral Tx erector spinae, contralateral transversospinalis
ROTATION	35-50°	Contralateral Tx erector spinae, ipsilateral transversospinalis

ORTHOPAEDIC TESTING OF THE THORACIC SPINE (TX)

Test 1: ADSON'S TEST

Why do we do the test?	To identify neurovascular compression - by the anterior scalene muscle and/or cervical rib - of the subclavian artery and the brachial plexus.
How do we do the test?	1. Have the client seated in front of you, with their supinated forearm resting on their thighs. 2. Working on the involved side, locate the client's radial pulse and determine its force and amplitude. 3. Instruct the client to turn their head to the involved side and elevate their chin and hold a deep breath
What you don't want to find?	That the pulse weakens or disappears, or the client's symptoms are reproduced.

Test 2: WRIGHT'S TEST

Why do we do the test?	To identify hyperabduction syndrome, which is compression of the axillary artery by the pectoralis minor muscle
How do we do the test?	1. Have the client seated in front of you. 2. Working on the involved side, locate the client's radial pulse and slowly abduct the client's arm to 180°
What you don't want to find?	That the pulse weakens or disappears, or the client's symptoms are reproduced

Test 3: COSTOCLAVICULAR TEST

Why do we do the test?	To identify Costoclavicular syndrome, which is neurovascular compression between the clavicle and the 1st rib
How do we do the test?	1. Have the client seated in front of you 2. Working on the involved side, locate the client's radial pulse and depress and push the shoulder posteriorly. 3. To reinforce the test, ask the client to flex the chin to chest.
What you don't want to find?	That the pulse weakens or disappears, or the client's symptoms are reproduced

	**Test 4: SLUMP TEST**
Why do we do the test?	The slump position increases the neural tension through traction of the spinal cord from above, either reproducing (aggravating) the client's symptoms or making the SLR test more sensitive.
How do we do the test?	1. Have the client seated in front of you at the edge of the table, with legs supported, the hips in a neutral position and the hands behind the back 2. Whilst keeping the chin and neck in a neutral posture, have the client 'slump' forward into thoracic and lumbar flexion. Apply pressure across the client's shoulders to maintain flexion of the thoracic and lumbar spines 3. Instruct the client to take their chin towards their chest. Apply additional pressure to the cervical region to maintain flexion of the cervical spine 4. Holding the client's foot in maximal dorsiflexion, have the client extend their knee as far as possible 5. Repeat the test on the other side
What you don't want to find?	Radicular pain
	**Test 5: RESPIRATORY RIB FUNCTION TEST**
Why do we do the test?	To assess for possible rib motion dysfunction during both inhalation and exhalation
How do we do the test?	1. Have the client seated or supine. 2. Place the hands in a relaxed fashion over the upper chest and hook finger tips over clavicle. This is to assess pump handle motion. 3. Move the hands down to the middle chest to assess for bucket handle motion. 4. Wrap the hands around the lower ribs to assess for the calliper motion.
What you don't want to find?	The rib motion not symmetrical from side to side or client reporting local pain and; if a rib stops moving relative to the other ribs during motion.

R.O.M.T OF THE (LX) LUMBAR SPINE

MOVEMENT	RANGE	KEY MUSCLES AFFECTED BY R.O.M
FLEXION	40-50°	Lx Erector spinae, multifidis, rotatores
EXTENSION	15-30°	Rectus abdominis, internal and external obliques, transverse abdominis
LATERAL FLEXION	25-35°	Contralateral quadartus lumborum, contralateral Lx erector spinae and contralateral transversospinalis
ROTATION	3-20°	Contralateral Lx erector spinae, ipsilateral transversospinalis

ORTHOPAEDIC TESTING OF THE THORACIC SPINE (TX)

Test 1: SLUMP TEST

Why do we do the test?	The slump position increases the neural tension through traction of the spinal cord from above, either reproducing (aggravating) the client's symptoms or making the SLR test more sensitive.
How do we do the test?	1. Have the client seated in front of you at the edge of the table, with legs supported, the hips in a neutral position and the hands behind the back 2. Whilst keeping the chin and neck in a neutral posture, have the client 'slump' forward into thoracic and lumbar flexion. Apply pressure across the client's shoulders to maintain flexion of the thoracic and lumbar spines 3. Instruct the client to take their chin towards their chest. Apply additional pressure to the cervical region to maintain flexion of the cervical spine 4. Holding the client's foot in maximal dorsiflexion, have the client extend their knee as far as possible 5. Repeat the test on the other side
What you don't want to find?	Radicular pain

Test 2: STRAIGHT LEG RAISE (SLR)

Why do we do the test?	This test is primarily used to detect nerve root irritation; if pain is radiating (neurogenic) then the possibilities are: 1. Space occupying lesion (eg. Disc protrusion or spinal tumour) 2. Piriformis Syndrome 3. Lumbar or SI joint dysfunction If the pain is local (thigh or low back), the possibilities include: 1. Hamstring strain 2. SI joint lesion 3. Hip joint lesion 4. Facet syndrome
How do we do the test?	1. Have the client supine on the table 2. Working with the involved leg, support the heel with one hand and place the other over the knee so as to prevent knee flexion 3. Slowly raise the leg toward 90° of hip flexion. Record the angle at which pain occurs as well as the site of pain

Special notes:	
If the test produces sciatic pain and if the foot is passively dorsiflexed and increases the pain, it is evidence of radiculopathy. Most of the movement during this test occurs at the L5 and S1 nerve root levels. The greatest tension occurs at 60-80°. When the limitation is 45° or less, then disc herniation must be strongly suspected. If pain is felt after about 70°, then look for other causes other than disc. If the client's knee flexes at any stage during the test, then this is a positive buckling sign and again strongly suggests sciatica of disc origin.	
What you don't want to find?	Radicular pain

Test 3: PRONE KNEE BEND (NACHLAS' TEST)	
Why do we do the test?	The test can indicate a lesion of the lumbosacral and /or SI joints if low back pain is produced, however if anterior thigh pain is noted, it can indicate femoral nerve involvement or a quadriceps strain.
How do we do the test?	1. Have the client prone on the table 2. Working on the involved side, flex the client's knee whilst stabilising the pelvis to prevent the hip from raising off the table
What you don't want to find?	Pain produced in the SI joint, lumbosacral joint or down the thigh and leg.

Test 4: QUADRANT TEST	
Why do we do the test?	**To produces maximum narrowing of the intervertebral foramen (IVF) and stress on the facet joints to the side which rotation occurs and also to assess for facet dysfunction**
How do we do the test?	1. Have the client standing in front of you. 2. Whilst holding the client's shoulders for support, instruct the client to extend the spine 3. Apply pressure in extension whilst the client side bends and rotates to the side of pain 4. The movement is continued until the limit of range is reached or until symptoms are produced
What you don't want to find?	Reproduction of the client's pain.

R.O.M.T OF THE HIP and THIGH

MOVEMENT	RANGE	KEY MUSCLES AFFECTED BY R.O.M
FLEXION	Flexed Knee- 120° Extended Knee- 90°	Hamstrings, gluteus maximus, adductor magnus
EXTENSION	0-15°	Rectus femoris, Iliopsoas
MEDIAL (INTERNAL) ROTATION	0-45°	Adductors, medial, hamstrings
EXTERNAL (LATERAL) ROTATION	0-30°	TFL, gluteus medius, minimus
ABDUCTION	0-40°	Piriformis and the deep external hip rotators
ADDUCTION	0-45°	TFL, gluteus minimus and gluteus medius

ORTHOPAEDIC TESTING OF THE HIP and THIGH

Test 1: SLUMP TEST

Why do we do the test?	The slump position increases the neural tension through traction of the spinal cord from above, either reproducing (aggravating) the client's symptoms or making the SLR test more sensitive.
How do we do the test?	1. Have the client seated in front of you at the edge of the table, with legs supported, the hips in a neutral position and the hands behind the back 2. Whilst keeping the chin and neck in a neutral posture, have the client 'slump' forward into thoracic and lumbar flexion. Apply pressure across the client's shoulders to maintain flexion of the thoracic and lumbar spines 3. Instruct the client to take their chin towards their chest. Apply additional pressure to the cervical region to maintain flexion of the cervical spine 4. Holding the client's foot in maximal dorsiflexion, have the client extend their knee as far as possible 5. Repeat the test on the other side
What you don't want to find?	Radicular pain

Test 2: STRAIGHT LEG RAISE (SLR)

Why do we do the test?	This test is primarily used to detect nerve root irritation; if pain is radiating (neurogenic) then the possibilities are: 1. Space occupying lesion (eg. Disc protrusion or spinal tumour) 2. Piriformis Syndrome 3. Lumbar or SI joint dysfunction If the pain is local (thigh or low back), the possibilities include: 1. Hamstring strain 2. SI joint lesion 3. Hip joint lesion 4. Facet syndrome
How do we do the test?	1. Have the client supine on the table 2. Working with the involved leg, support the heel with one hand and place the other over the knee so as to prevent knee flexion 3. Slowly raise the leg toward 90° of hip flexion. Record the angle at which pain occurs as well as the site of pain

Special notes:	
	If the test produces sciatic pain and if the foot is passively dorsiflexed and increases the pain, it is evidence of radiculopathy. Most of the movement during this test occurs at the L5 and S1 nerve root levels. The greatest tension occurs at 60-80°. When the limitation is 45° or less, then disc herniation must be strongly suspected. If pain is felt after about 70°, then look for other causes other than disc. If the client's knee flexes at any stage during the test, then this is a positive buckling sign and again strongly suggests sciatica of disc origin.
What you don't want to find?	Radicular pain

Test 3: PRONE KNEE BEND (NACHLAS' TEST)

Why do we do the test?	The test can indicate a lesion of the lumbosacral and /or SI joints if low back pain is produced, however if anterior thigh pain is noted, it can indicate femoral nerve involvement or a quadriceps strain.
How do we do the test?	1. Have the client prone on the table 2. Working on the involved side, flex the client's knee whilst stabilising the pelvis to prevent the hip from raising off the table
What you don't want to find?	Pain produced in the SI joint, lumbosacral joint or down the thigh and leg.

Test 4: THOMAS TEST

Why do we do the test?	To test for Iliopsoas and/or rectus femoris shortness
How do we do the test?	Have the client lie supine on the table with their buttocks (coccyx) as close to the edge of table as possible. Holding the non-involved leg at the knee in hip and knee flexion (full flexion of the hip helps to maintain the pelvis in full rotation with the lumbar spine flat, which is essential if the test is to be meaningful and stress on the spine is to be avoided).
What you don't want to find?	1. Suspect Iliopsoas shortness if the thigh of the involved leg cannot be extended to be horizontal, parallel with the table 2. Suspect rectus femoris shortness if the lower part of the involved leg cannot be flexed to achieve almost 90° angle with the thigh

Test 5: OBER'S TEST

Why do we do the test?	To test for TFL (tensor fascia latae) shortness
How do we do the test?	1. Standing behind the client, have them lie on table with their back close to the edge of the table, lower leg flexed at the hip and knee for stability. 2. Support the client's top leg at the ankle and knee and ensure there is no hip flexion, which would nullify the test. 3. Carefully flex the client's knee to 90°, without allowing the hip to flex. Then - supporting just the ankle, allow the knee to fall towards the table. 4. If TFL is normal, the thigh and knee will fall easily, with the knee contacting the table surface (unless unusual hip width, or thigh length prevent this) 5. If the upper leg remains aloft, with little sign of 'falling' towards the table, then either the client is not letting go or the TFL is short and does not allow it to fall. As a rule, the band will palpate as tender under such conditions

Test 6: SHORT QUADRICEPS TEST	
Why do we do the test?	To test for Short Quadriceps
How do we do the test?	1. Standing beside the table, have the client lie prone, ideally with a cushion under the abdomen to avoid hyperlordosis
2. With one hand over the sacral area to stabilise the pelvis, hold the lower leg with your other hand and flex the knee of the client
3. If Rectus femoris is short, then the client's heel will not easily be able to touch the buttock
Test 7: HAMSTRING LENGTH TEST	
Why do we do the test?	To test for shortness of hamstring muscles
How do we do the test?	1. Have the client supine on the table with non-involved leg either flexed or straight, depending on previous test results for hip flexors
2. Standing beside the client facing towards the head of the table, gently take the involved leg into a straight leg raised position with an extended knee
3. The first sign of resistance (or palpated bind) is assessed as the barrier of restriction
4. Suspect shortening of the hamstrings if a straight leg raise to 80° is not easily possible
5. The muscles can be treated in the straight leg position
Test 8: LONG ADDUCTORS vs SHORT ADDUCTORS TEST	
Why do we do the test?	To test shortness of adductors
How do we do the test?	1. Standing beside the table, have the client lie supine. Abduct the leg to its easy barrier and then flex the knee
2. If - after knee flexion has been introduced - further abduction is easily achieved, suspect that any previous limitation to abduction was the result of medial hamstring shortness, since this is no longer operating once the knee has been flexed.
3. If, however, restriction remains, suspect that the short adductors are continuing to prevent movement and are in a shortened position.
Test 9: PIRIFORMIS STRETCH TEST	
Why do we do the test?	To test for a shortened piriformis
How do we do the test?	1. When short, the piriformis muscle will cause the involved leg to appear short and externally rotated when the client is supine
2. Standing beside the table, have the client lie supine
3. Flex the hip and knee of the involved leg and place the foot across the non-involved leg to rest on the table. The angle of hip flexion should not exceed 60°. This position should cause a stretch of the shortened piriformis muscle

R.O.M.T OF THE KNEE		
MOVEMENT	RANGE	KEY MUSCLES AFFECTED BY R.O.M
FLEXION	0-135°	Quadriceps, TFL (0-30° of flexion)
EXTENSION	0-15°	Hamstrings, gracilis, gastrocnemius, popliteus, plantaris, TFL (in 45-145° of flextion
MEDIAL (INTERNAL) ROTATION	20-30°	Biceps Femoris (non-weight bearing)
LATERAL (EXTERNAL) ROTATION	30-40°	Popliteus, semimembranosus, semitendinosus, Sartorius, gracilis (non- weight)

ORTHOPAEDIC TESTING OF THE KNEE

TEST 1: VALGUS / VARUS STRESS TEST

Valgus Stress	If the test is positive with the knee in extension, the following structures may have been injured to some degree:
1. Medial collateral ligament 2. Posterior oblique ligament 3. Posteromedial capsule	4. Anterior cruciate ligament 5. Medial quadriceps expansion 6. Semimembranosus muscle
Varus Stress	If the test is positive with the knee in extension, the following structures may have been injured to some degree:
1. Lateral collateral ligament 2. Posterolateral capsule 3. Arcuate-popliteal complex	4. Biceps femoris tendon 7. Iliotibial band 5. Anterior cruciate ligament 6. Lateral gastrocnemius muscle
How do we do the test?	Have the client supine on the table with the knees extended. Working on the involved side, stabilise the foot on the table and push the knee into valgum and varum positions alternatively.
What you don't want to find?	Excessive Motion

TEST 2: ANTEROPOSTERIOR DRAWER TEST

For anterior drawer test, normal translator motion of the tibia on the femur is approximately 6mm. If excessive motion (greater than 6mm) is found, the following structures may have been injured to some degree:

1. Anterior cruciate ligament
2. Posterolateral capsule
3. Posteromedial capsule
4. Medial collateral ligament
5. Iliotibial band
6. Posterior oblique ligament
7. Arcuate-popliteus complex

If excessive motion is found on the posterior drawer test, the following structures may have been injured to some degree:

1. Posterior cruciate ligament
2. Arcuate-popliteus complex
3. Posterior oblique ligament
4. Anterior cruciate ligament

How do we do the test?	1. Have the client supine on the table, with the involved leg in 75-90° of knee flexion. 2. Seated on the table -with your hip stabilising and fixing the client's foot - firmly grasp the proximal leg with both hands and apply alternating anterior and posterior stress.
What you don't want to find?	Excessive movement in an anterior or posterior direction (this is a positive sign)

Test 3: McMURRAY'S CLICK TEST	
Why do we do the test?	To assess for medial or lateral meniscal lesions
How do we do the test?	To test the medial meniscus:
1. Have the client supine on the table with the knee and hip flexed so that the heel of the foot is close to the buttock 2. Standing on the involved side, place your cephalad hand over the client's knee and grasp their foot with your caudal hand (have the fingers of the cephalad hand over the medial joint space and the thumb over the lateral joint space) 3. Pull the knee into abduction (valgus stress) with the foot and leg in extern.al rotation 4. Extend the knee whilst holding it in strong abduction	
How do we do the test?	To test the lateral meniscus:
1. Have the client supine on the table with the knee and hip flexed so that the heel of the foot is close to the buttock. 2. Standing on the involved side, place your cephalad hand over the client's knee and grasp their foot with your caudal hand (have the fingers of the cephalad hand over the medial joint space and the thumb over the lateral joint space). 3. Pull the knee into adduction (varus stress) with the foot and leg in medial rotation 4. Extend the knee whilst holding it in strong adduction	
What you don't want to find?	If there are loose fragments of the lateral meniscus (or medial meniscus), the action may cause a snap or click that is often accompanied by pain
Test 4: APLEY'S GRIND AND DISTRACTION TEST	
Why do we do the test?	**The compression component of the test assesses for meniscal damage, the distraction component of the test assesses for non-specific ligament damage.**
How do we do the test?	1. Have the client prone on the table with the involved knee flexed to 90° 2. Stabilise the thigh by pressing down firmly, but gently, with either hand or knee (required mainly for the distraction component), and grasp the client's foot. 3. Apply downward pressure to the foot to compress the medial and lateral menisci between the tibia and femur 4. Internally and externally rotate the tibia on the femur while maintaining downward pressure 5. Then apply distraction with the ankle, again internally and externally rotating the tibia
What you don't want to find?	On compression - pain or crepitation; on distraction - pain or laxity.
Test 5: PATELLOFEMORAL GRINDING TEST (FOUCHET'S SIGN)	
Why do we do the test?	To assess for patellofemoral pain syndrome (chondromalacia patellae).
How do we do the test?	1. Have the client supine on the table with the involved knee extended 2. Using the web of the hand, apply downward pressure just proximal to the base of the patella 3. Ask the client to contract the quadriceps muscles whilst you push down
What you don't want to find?	If the test causes retro patellar pain and the client cannot hold a contraction, the test is considered positive.

Test 6: PATELLAR APPREHENSION TEST	
Why do we do the test?	To assess for recurrent patellar dislocation
How do we do the test?	1. Have the client supine on the table with the involved knee extended 2. Using both hands, grasp above and below the patella, and use your thumbs to push the patella laterally (this test can also be performed with the knee flexed at 30°)
What you don't want to find?	The test is considered positive if the client stops you from moving the patellar any further.

R.O.M.T OF THE ANKLE		
MOVEMENT	RANGE	KEY MUSCLES AFFECTED BY R.O.M
PLANTARFLEXION	0-50°	Tibialis anterior, extensor hallicus longus, extensor digitorum longus
DORSIFLEXION	10-20°	Soleus (flexed Knee), gastrocnemius (Knee extended)
INVERSION	45-60°	Peroneus longus, peroneus brevis, extensor digitorum longus
EVERSION	15-30°	Tibialis anterior, tibialis posterior, flexor digitorum longus, flexor hallicus longus, extensor hallicus longus

ORTHOPAEDIC TESTING OF THE ANKLE

Test 1: THOMSON'S TEST

Why do we do the test?	To assess for a complete rupture of the Achilles tendon
How do we do the test?	1. Have the client prone on the table, with their feet off the end of the table 2. Squeeze the calf muscle; this should cause slight plantar flexion of the ankle
What you don't want to find?	This test is considered positive if the ankle does not plantar flex.

Test 2: ANTERIOR FOOT DRAWER TEST

Why do we do the test?	To assess for a tear of the anterior talofibular ligament.
How do we do the test?	1. Have the client supine with feet relaxed. 2. Stabilising the anterior aspect of the ankle with one hand and grasping the calcaneus with the other, push the tibia posteriorly whilst drawing the calcaneus anteriorly (normally there should be no anterior movement).
What you don't want to find?	This test is considered positive if the talus slides anteriorly

Test 3: ANKLE LATERAL AND MEDIAL STABILITY TEST

Why do we do the test?	To assess for damage to the distal, anterior and posterior tibiofibular ligaments. The deltoid may also be involved (along with - possibly- the interosseous membrane).
How do we do the test?	1. Have the client supine with feet relaxed. 2. Holding onto the heel of the involved foot, produce inversion and eversion stress
What you don't want to find?	This test is considered positive if rocking of the talus is produced

R.O.M.T OF THE SHOULDER		
MOVEMENT	RANGE	KEY MUSCLES AFFECTED BY R.O.M
FLEXION	0-180°	Latissimus Dorsi, teres major, sternocostal fibres of pec major, posterior deltoid
EXTENSION	0-50°	Clavicular fibres of pec major, anterior deltoid, biceps brachii
ABDUCTION	0-180°	Latissimus dorsi, teres major, pectoralis (pec) major
ADDUCTION	0-50°	Supraspinatus, deltoid
INTERNAL ROTATION	0-90°	Infraspinatus, teres minor, posterior deltoid
EXTERNAL ROTATION	0-90°	Subscapularis, latissimus dorsi, teres mojor, pec major, anterior deltoid
HORIZONTAL FLEXION (ADDUCTION)	0-140°	Infraspinatus, teres minor, posterior deltoid
HORIZONTAL EXTENTION (ABDUCTION)	0-40°	Pectoralis (pec) major, anterior deltoid

Test 1: PECTORALIS MAJOR vs LATISSIMUS DORSI TEST

Why do we do the test?	To find out if the client has a hypertonic latissimus dorsi or pectoral is major.
How do we do the test?	1. We place the client in a supine position and move them down the table a little bit with both hips and knees flexed and their feet resting on the table. 2. We get them to flex both arms above the head and let them rest on the table completely relaxed. 3. Now we observe the arm positions and if everything is normal, the elbows should rest on the table close to the ears
What you don't want to find?	If pectoralis major is dysfunctional, the elbow will rest off the table because it is held in an extended position by the muscle. If latissimus dorsi is dysfunctional, the elbow will rest away from the ears in an adducted position by the muscle.

Test 2: LATISSIMUS DORSI TRUNK FLEXION TEST

Why do we do the test?	To find out if the client's latissimus dorsi is short or has a dysfunction
How do we do the test?	1. Ask the standing client to flex the torso and bend forwards so their torso is parallel with the floor (half-bent position). Have them allow the arms to freely hang from the shoulders. 2. From here, the therapist stands in front of the client (who remains half-bent). 3. While stabilising the scapula with one hand, the therapist grasps the arm just proximal to the elbow and gently draws the straight arm forward.
What you don't want to find?	If there is not excessive 'bind' in the tissues being tested, the arm should easily reach a level higher than the back of the head. If not possible, then latissimus dorsi is short.

Test 3: SUBSCAPULARIS/PECTORALIS MINOR TEST	
Why do we do the test?	To find out if the client has a hypertonic subscapularis or pectoralis minor.
How do we do the test?	1. We place the client in a supine position with the shoulder abducted to 90° and elbow flexed to 90° with the palm pronated and facing the feet. 2. We get them to let their hand fall back towards the floor so their palm should be now pointed towards the ceiling. 3. Now we observe the arm position and if everything is normal the forearm should be lying parallel to the floor.
What you don't want to find?	A forearm that is unable to lie parallel with the floor tells us that subscapularis or pectoralis minor is dysfunctional. If the shoulder appears to be protracted then it is almost always pectoral is minor that is the cause.
Test 4: APLEY'S SCRATCH TEST	
Why do we do the test?	To find out if the client has restricted ROM in any of the following positions: lateral rotation, flexion, abduction, medial rotation, extension and adduction or any signs of capsular restriction.
How do we do the test?	Have the client take their right arm into abduction, bend the arm and try to reach their C7 vertebrae with their fingers. Then take their left hand behind their back and try to touch their other hand.
What you don't want to find?	Any pain, hypertonicity or excessive restriction in the general ROM.
Test 5: SHOULDER ABDUCTION TEST (BAKODY'S)	
Why do we do the test?	To test for radicular symptoms, especially those involving C4 or C5 nerve roots.
How do we do the test?	The client is sitting or lying supine and the therapist passively abducts the arm until the forearm rests on top of the client's head.
What you don't want to find?	A decrease or relief of the symptoms can indicate a cervical extradural compression problem such as a herniated disc or nerve root compression.
Test 6: THE LIFT-OFF TEST	
Why do we do the test?	To test the integrity of the subscapularis muscle.
How do we do the test?	1. The client stands and places the back of the hand on the back or against the mid lumbar spine. 2. The client then lifts the hand away from the back. An inability to do so indicates a lesion of subscapularis muscle 3. Abnormal motion in the scapula during the test may indicate scapular instability. 4. If the client is able to take the hand away from the back, the therapist should apply a load, pushing the hand toward the back to test the strength of the subscapularis and to test how the scapula acts under dynamic load
What you don't want to find?	Subscapularis is found to be weak if the client's hand moves towards the back after lift-off, or there is any pain.

ORTHOPAEDIC TESTS OF THE SHOULDER

Test 1: NEER IMPINGEMENT TEST

Why do we do the test?	To determine whether there is an overuse injury in the supraspinatus muscle or sometimes the tendon of the long head of the biceps brachii muscle.
How do we do the test?	1. Have the client seated in front of you at the edge of the table. 2. Holding the client's arm to support the elbow, passively and forcibly move the client's arm into full abduction then medial rotation. This passive movement causes jamming of the greater tubercle against the anteroinferior border of the acromion.
What you don't want to find?	Pain displayed on the client's face or any verbal displays of pain.

Test 2: HAWKINS-KENNEDY IMPINGEMENT TEST

Why do we do the test?	To ascertain if there is any impingement of the supraspinatus tendon against the coracoacromial ligament and also to detect the presence of any crepitus at the subacromial bursa.
How do we do the test?	1. Have the client seated facing you at the edge of the table. 2. Have the client place their arm in a throw follow through position and flexed forward to 30° 3. Holding the client's arm at the elbow, passively and forcibly move the client's shoulder into medial rotation. This passive movement pushes the supraspinatus tendon against the anterior surface of the coracoacromial ligament and the coracoid process.
What you don't want to find?	Pain displayed on the client's face or any verbal displays of pain.

Test 3: POSTERIOR INTERNAL IMPINGEMENT TEST

Why do we do the test?	To indicate an impingement between the rotator cuff and the greater tubercle plus the posterior glenoid and the labrum.
How do we do the test?	1. Have the client supine on the table. 2. Holding the client's arm to support the elbow and the wrist, passively abduct the shoulder to 90° with approximately 15-20° of forward flexion and maximal lateral rotation
What you don't want to find?	Localised pain in the posterior shoulder

Test 4: EMPTY CAN OR JOBE'S TEST (SUPRASPINATUS TEST)

Why do we do the test?	To indicate any weakness and pain that would indicate a tear or inflammation of the supraspinatus tendon or muscle. In the normal functioning shoulder, the subacromial space severely decreases when the shoulder is between 45 and 160°. A swollen and inflamed tendon would cause pain through this range.
How do we do the test?	1. Have the client seated facing you at the edge of the table. 2. Whilst applying resistance, have the client abduct the shoulders to 90°. 3. Passively medially rotate the shoulders and angle them forward with the client's thumbs pointing towards the floor. Ask the client to abduct as we again resist abduction.
What you don't want to find?	If the client exhibits weakness or experiences pain then the test is positive

	Test 5: ACROMIOCLAVICULAR SHEAR TEST
Why do we do the test?	To assess for any acromioclavicular joint pathology such as arthritis.
How do we do the test?	1. Have the client seated facing you at the edge of the table 2. Cup your hands over the deltoid muscle, with one hand on the clavicle and one hand on the spine of the scapula 3. Squeeze the heels of the hands together
What you don't want to find?	Pain or abnormal movement indicates a positive test.
	Test 6: LOAD AND SHIFT TEST
Why do we do the test?	To assess atraumatic instability problems of the GH (GLENOHUMERAL) joint
How do we do the test?	1. Have the client seated in front of you at the edge of the table in ideal posture, with the hand of the affected arm resting on the thigh 2. Stand behind the client and stabilise the shoulder with one hand over the clavicle and scapula. The other hand grasps the head of the humerus with the thumb over the posterior humeral head and the fingers over the anterior humeral head 3. Run the fingers along the anterior humerus and the thumb along the posterior humerus to 'feel'; where the humerus is seated relative to the glenoid. If the fingers 'dip in' anteriorly as they move medially, but the thumb does not, it indicates the humeral head is sitting anteriorly. Normally, the humeral head feels a little bit more anteriorly when it is seated in the glenoid 4. Protraction of the scapula causes the glenoid head to shift anteriorly in the glenoid. The therapist must be careful with the finger and thumb placement so as not to cause pain 5. The humerus is then pushed anteriorly or posteriorly in the glenoid if necessary to 'seat' it properly in the glenoid fossa. This places the head of the humerus in its normal position relative to the glenoid. This is the 'load' portion of the test. If load is not applied, there is no normal starting position 6. Push the humeral head anteriorly or posteriorly and note the amount of translation and end feel (this is the shift portion). A false negative test can occur with anterior translation if the head is not centred 7. Repeat the test on the other side
What you don't want to find?	Translation greater than 25%

R.O.M.T OF THE WRIST and ELBOW			
MOVEMENT	RANGE	KEY MUSCLES AFFECTED BY R.O.M
ELBOW FLEXION	140-150°	Triceps Brachii, Anconeus
ELBOW EXTENTION	0-10°	Biceps Brachii, Brachialis, Brachioradialis
FOREARM PRONATION	80-90°	Pronator Teres
FOREARM SUPERNATION	80-90°	Supinator, Biceps Brachii
WRIST FLEXION	80-90°	Common Extensors
WRIST EXTENTION	70-90°	Common flexors
ORTHOPAEDIC TESTS		
Test 1: COZENS TEST		
Why do we do the test?	To find out if the client has extensor tendinopathy	
How do we do the test?	1. Have the client seated facing you 2. Support the client's elbow from underneath with a cupped hand, your thumb on the lateral epicondyle and your fingers on the medial condyle 3. Instruct the client to make a fist, then - have the client pronate the forearm and radially deviate and extend the wrist - resist wrist extension	
What you don't want to find?	If there is a sudden severe pain in the area of the lateral epicondyle we can consider the test positive	
Test 2: MILL'S TEST		
Why do we do the test?	To find out if the client has extensor tendinopathy	
How do we do the test?	1. Have the client seated facing you 2. Support the client's elbow from underneath with a cupped hand, your thumb on the lateral epicondyle and your fingers on the medial condyle 3. Instruct the client to make a fist, then pronate the forearm and fully flex the wrist whilst extending the elbow	
What you don't want to find?	A positive result would be achieved if there is pain at the lateral epicondyle	
Test 3: LATERAL EPICONDYLE EXTENSION TEST		
Why do we do the test?	To find out if the client has extensor tendinopathy	
How do we do the test?	1. Have the client seated facing you 2. Instruct the client to hold their hand out with the forearm pronated, palm facing downwards 3. Using your first two fingers, apply resistance to the client's middle digit as they extend the finger (this places strain on the extensor digitorum muscle and tendon)	
What you don't want to find?	A positive result would be achieved if there is pain at the lateral epicondyle	

Test 4: FLEXOR/PRONATOR TENDINOPATHY TEST	
Why do we do the test?	To find out if the client has flexor/pronator tendinopathy
How do we do the test?	1. Have the client seated facing you 2. Whilst supporting the client's arm, passively supinate the forearm and extend the elbow and wrist as you palpate their medial epicondyle
What you don't want to find?	If there is pain over the medial epicondyle we can consider the test positive

Test 5: TINEL'S SIGN (AT THE ELBOW)	
Why do we do the test?	To determine the point of regeneration of sensory nerve fibres (the most distal point at which the abnormal sensation is felt represents the limit of nerve regeneration)
How do we do the test?	1. Have the client seated facing you 2. Whilst supporting the client's arm, tap the area around the ulnar nerve with your finger (this is the area in the groove between the olecranon process and the medial epicondyle)
What you don't want to find?	A positive result is indicated by a tingling sensation in the ulnar distribution of the forearm and the hand distal to the point of compression of the nerve

Test 6: PHALEN'S TEST	
Why do we do the test?	To find out if the client has carpal tunnel syndrome
How do we do the test?	1. Have the client seated facing you 2. Instruct the client to flex both wrists to 90 degrees by bringing the back of the hands together and holding this position for 60 seconds (in carpal tunnel syndrome this exacerbates or reproduces the symptoms)
What you don't want to find?	A positive test is indicated by tingling in the thumb, index finger and middle and lateral half of the ring finger

	**Test 7: TINEL'S SIGN**
Why do we do the test?	To find out if the client has carpal tunnel syndrome
How do we do the test?	1. Have the client seated facing you with their supinated arm and hand resting on the table 2. Using your fingers, tap over the pal mar surface of the wrist (this precipitates pain in the median nerve distribution)
What you don't want to find?	A positive test causes tingling or paraesthesia into the thumb, index finger and middle and lateral half of the ring finger
	**Test 8: CARPAL COMPRESSION TEST**
Why do we do the test?	To find out if the client has carpal tunnel syndrome
How do we do the test?	1. Have the client seated facing you with their supinated arm and hand resting on the table 2. Hold the client's wrist in both hands, apply direct pressure over the median nerve in the carpal tunnel for up to 30 seconds
What you don't want to find?	A positive result would be achieved if the client's usual pain is reproduced
	**Test 9: FINKELSTEIN'S TEST**
Why do we do the test?	To find out if the client has De Quervain's disease
How do we do the test?	1. Have the client seated facing you with their hand in a fist, with the thumb inside the fingers 2. While stabilising the forearm with one hand, use the other hand to deviate the wrist towards the ulnar side
What you don't want to find?	A positive result would be achieved if the client feels pain over the abductor pollicis longus and extensor pollicis longus tendons at the wrist

ABBREVIATIONS

Clinical Terms	
ABBREVIATIONS	MEANING
ADL	Activities of daily living
AMC	Abnormal muscle contraction
TP/ TrP	Trigger point
MPS	Myofascial pain syndrome
Abn	Abnormal
Adh	Adhesion
ROM	Range of movement
GOM	Grade of contraction
o/ e	On examination
CC	Chief complaint
c/ o	Complains of
Hx	History
PH	Past history
Dx	Diagnosis
WDx	Working diagnosis
DDx	Differential diagnosis
Rx	Treatment
P, p, Ⓟ	Pain
mm	Muscle/ muscles
R	Right
L	Left
BP	Blood pressure
LOC	Loss of consciousness
SOB	Shortness of breath
MVA	Motor vehicle accident
MvT	Movement
Jnt	Joint
Cx	Cervical
Tx	Thoracic
Lx	Lumbar
Bi	Bilateral
Uni	Unilateral
s & s	Signs & symptoms

NOTES

Clinical Terms	
ABBREVIATIONS	MEANING
W	With
W/O	Without
Fxn	Function
H.R.	Heart rate
Rxn	Reaction
N (WITH CIRCLE AROUND IT)	Normal
n/ nn	Nerve/ nerves
Mx	Massage treatment
Fx/ FxHx	Family history
d/t	Due to
b/w	Between
a/ aa	Artery/ arteries
POST	Posterior
ANT	Anterior
lig.	Ligament
MVA	Motor vehicle accident
R/T or r/t	Related to

SYMBOLS	
SYMBOL	MEANING
<	Less than
>	Greater than
~	Approximately
1/60	One minute
1/24	One hour
1/7	One day
1/52	One week
1/12	One month
↑	Increase
↓	Decrease
#/ F	Fracture
∴ OR ∴	Therefore
♀	Female
♂	Male

MOVEMENT TERMS

ABBREVIATIONS	MEANING
Add	Adduction
Abd	Abduction
Ext	Extension
Flex	Flexion
Sup	Supination
Pron	Pronation
D/ Flex	Dorsiflexion
P/ Flex	Plantar flexion
L/ Rot	Lateral rotation
M/ Rot	Medial rotation
R/ Dev	Radial deviation
U/ Dev	Ulnar deviation

TREATMENT TERMS

ABBREVIATIONS	MEANING
STM	Soft tissue manipulation, superficial therapeutic massage
DTM	Deep tissue/ therapeutic massage
TM	Therapeutic massage
MT	Mobilising therapy
MFR	Myofascial release
MfC	Myofascial cupping
TENS	Transcutaneous electronic nerve stimulation
PNF	Proprioceptive neuromuscular facilitation
DN	Dry needling
TT	Thermal therapies
HTx	Heat therapy
CTx	Cryotherapy
M/ STr	Myofascial stretch
I/ Com	Ischaemic compression

CARDIAC TERMS

ABBREVIATIONS	MEANING
VF	Ventricular fibrillation
AF	Atrial fibrillation
CCF	Congestive Cardiac failure

MEDICAL CONDITIONS

ABBREVIATIONS	MEANING
OA	Osteoarthritis
RA	Rheumatoid arthritis
MS	Multiple sclerosis
AS	Atherosclerosis
HBP	High blood pressure
LBP	Low blood pressure
IH	Infectious hepatitis
AIDS	Acquired immuno deficiency syndrome
HIV	Human immuno-deficiency virus
VBI	Vertebral basilar insufficiency
H/ah	Headache
FMS	Fibromyalgia syndrome
MPS	Myofascial pain syndrome

MUSCLE & LANDMARKS

ABBREVIATIONS	MEANING
Psis	Posterior superior iliac spine
Asis	Anterior superior iliac spine
Aiis	Anterior Inferior Iliac Spine
SCM	Sternocleidomastoid
ITB	Iliotibial band
Pec/Pecs	Pectoralis
TFL	Tensor Fascia Latae

NOTES

REFERENCES

- Lecture notes (Sage Institute of Education)
- SIM_AssessmentandOrthopaedicTests_1511_V1.0 (Sage Institute of Education)
- Consultant: James Wyatt (2016)

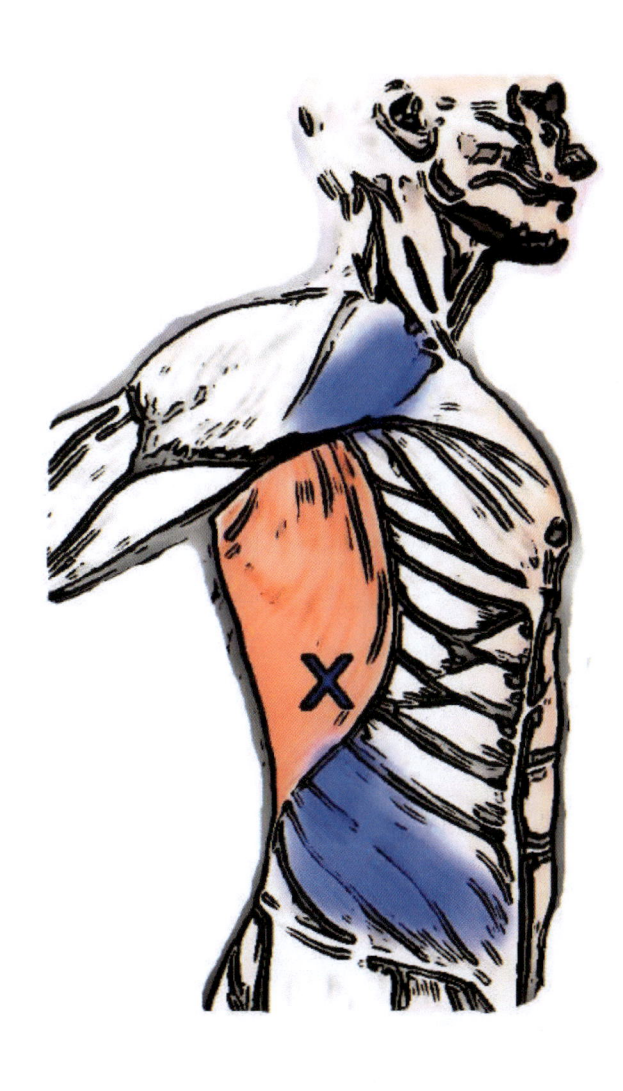

ILLUSTRATIONS BY

DANIEL THOMAS

Printed in Great Britain
by Amazon